Assessing the Support Needs of Adopted Children and Their Families

Building secure new lives

Liza Bingley Miller and
Arnon Bentovim

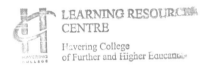
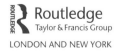
Routledge
Taylor & Francis Group

LONDON AND NEW YORK

First published 2007 by Routledge
2 Park Square, Milton Park, Abingdon, Oxon OX14 4RN

Simultaneously published in the USA and Canada
by Routledge
270 Madison Ave, New York, NY 10016

Routledge is an imprint of the Taylor & Francis Group, an informa business

© 2007 Liza Bingley Miller and Arnon Bentovim

Typeset in Times New Roman by
Florence Production Ltd, Stoodleigh, Devon
Printed and bound in Great Britain by
TJ International, Padstow, Cornwall

British Library Cataloguing in Publication Data
A catalogue record for this book is available from the British Library

Library of Congress Cataloging in Publication Data
Miller, Liza Bingley.
    Assessing the support needs of adopted children and their families: building
    secure placements – new lives/Liza Bingley Miller and Arnon Bentovim.
        p. cm.
        Includes bibliographical references and index.
    1. Adopted children–Great Britain.   2. Adoption–Great Britain.   3. Adoptive
    parents–Great Britain.   4. Adoptive parents–Services for–Great Britain.
    I. Bentovim, Arnon.   II. Title.
    HV875.58.G7M55 2006
    362.734–dc22   2006018387

ISBN10: 0–415–40944–6 (hbk)
ISBN10: 0–415–40945–4 (pbk)
ISBN10: 0–203–96519–1 (ebk)

ISBN13: 978–0–415–40944–5 (hbk)
ISBN13: 978–0–415–40945–2 (pbk)
ISBN13: 978–0–203–96519–1 (ebk)

Assessing the Support Needs of Adopted Children and Their Families

Every child deserves the chance to grow up in a stable, loving family and adoption offers children a crucial route to stability and security when they cannot live with their birth families. *Assessing the Support Needs of Adopted Children and their Families* looks at how effective support can help adoptive families respond to children's developmental needs, deal with stress and prevent placement breakdowns.

Written in consultation with a range of experts, clinicians and practitioners as well as adoptive children, families and birth relatives, *Assessing the Support Needs of Adopted Children and their Families* gives guidance on making evidence-based assessments and planning successful adoption support. Key features include:

- discussion of the main themes of adoption and pointers for practice in relation to the *Assessment Framework*;
- a guide to the use of evidence-based approaches to assessment, including the tools commissioned by the Department of Health and the Department for Education and Skills;
- a model for analysis and planning, and planning support and interventions; and
- investigation of the source, range and value of support services and interventions that can promote the wellbeing of adopted children, their adoptive families and birth relatives.

Packed with practical advice, case examples and models of good practice, this book is invaluable for social workers and managers involved with the adoption process and the wellbeing of children and families. It is also essential reading for social work students learning about working with children and families.

Liza Bingley Miller is the National Training Coordinator of the Child and Family Training Programme in Evidence-based approaches to Assessing Children and their Families. She also works at the University of York and is Chair of two Adoption Panels in North Yorkshire.

Arnon Bentovim is a child and family psychiatrist who worked for many years as a consultant at Great Ormond Street Children's Hospital and the Tavistock Clinic. He currently directs the London Child and Family Consultation Service and is an Honorary Senior Lecturer at the Institute of Child Health, University College London.

Contents

Acknowledgements

Liza Bingley Miller and Arnon Bentovim would like to thank the following professionals for their contribution to the development of this book. We would also like to thank members of the adoptive and birth families who contributed anonymously for their invaluable assistance in keeping a focus on adopted children and their families.

Margaret Adcock, Department of Child and Adolescent Mental Health, Great Ormond Street Hospital for Children, London.

Erica Amende, Director, Central and Northern Region, British Association for Adoption and Fostering (BAAF).

Hedi Argent, Independent Adoption Consultant, Trainer and Freelance Writer, London.

Melanie Atkins, Team Leader, Adopt Anglia, Cambridge.

Mary Beek, Senior Research Associate, Centre for Research on the Child and Family, University of East Anglia, Norwich.

Caroline Bengo, Adoption and Fostering Clinic, Maudsley Hospital, London.

Felicity Collier, Chief Executive, British Association for Adoption and Fostering.

Jonathan Corbett, Social Services Inspectorate for Wales.

Antony Cox, Emeritus Professor of Child and Adolescent Psychiatry, Guy's, King's and St Thomas' Hospital Schools of Medicine.

Maureen Crank, After Adoption, Manchester.

Wes Cuell, Director, Luton Social Services Department.

Rhonwyn Dobbing, Social Services Inspectorate for Wales.

Monica Duck, Director of the Post Adoption Centre, London.

George Eddon, Principal Lawyer (Children), North Yorkshire County Council.

Danya Glaser, Consultant Child and Adolescent Psychiatrist, Great Ormond Street Hospital for Children, London.

Sue Gourvish, Director, Fostering Network, London.

Marianne Halliday, Head of Adoption Support Team, Norfolk Social Services Department, Norwich.

Anthea Hendry, Art Psychotherapist, Child and Adolescent Mental Health Service, Leeds.

Jill Hodges, Consultant Child Psychotherapist, Great Ormond Street Hospital for Children, London.

Gail Jackson, Senior Practitioner Adoption Support, Catholic Children's Society, Nottingham.

Carol Jolliffe, Family Therapist, Child and Adolescent Mental Health Services (CAMHS), Kent.

Jeanne Kaniuk, Head of Coram Adoption Service, London.

Caroline Lindsey, Consultant Child Psychiatrist, Child and Family Department, Tavistock Clinic, London.

Ruth McCullum, Family Support Development Manager, Parents for Children.

Mary McKelvey, Service Manager, Family Placement, City of York Council.

Lyndsey Marshall, Manager, After Adoption Yorkshire, Leeds.

Judith Matthews, Leeds Social Services.

Elizabeth Monck, Thomas Coram Research Unit, London.

Elsbeth Neil, School of Social Work and Psychosocial Sciences, University of East Anglia, Norwich.

Mo O'Reilly, Adoption Agency Manager, Barnardos UK.

Jonathan Pearce, Director, Adoption UK, Banbury, Oxfordshire.

Stephen Pizzey, Social Work Consultant and Children's Guardian, Surrey.

Beverley Prevatt Goldstein, Black Ethnic Minority Community Organisations' Network (BECON), Newcastle upon Tyne.

Elaine Rose, Children's Guardian and Psychotherapist, Kent.

Brigid Sheehan, Social Worker, Adoption Team, Croydon Social Services.

John Simmonds, Director of Policy, Research and Development, British Association for Adoption and Fostering.

Margaret Staples, Principal Team Manager, Adoption Services, Nottinghamshire County Council.

Miriam Steele, Director, Anna Freud Clinic, London.

Cathy Stubbs, Adoption Team Manager, Reading Social Services.

Simon Tapp, Children's Guardian and Independent Social Worker, Kent.

Katrina Wilson, Information Officer, British Association for Adoption and Fostering, London.

Introduction

Context

Every child deserves the chance to grow up in a stable, loving family.
(Department of Health (DoH) 2002b)

Adoption and special guardianship offer children a crucial route to stability and security when they cannot live with their birth families, for whatever reason. Effective adoption and special guardianship support is important in helping families respond to children's developmental needs, to deal with stress and to prevent placement breakdowns wherever possible (Fratter et al. 1991; Lowe 1997, 2000; Selwyn and Quinton 2004; Thoburn 1990; Ward 2004).

This book looks at the assessment of the support needs of adopted children and their families including the following:

- Children placed for adoption and their prospective adoptive families.
- Adopted children and their adoptive families.
- Children cared for under special guardianship orders, the special guardians and their families.
- Birth families in relation to facilitating contact and the needs of their children who have been placed for adoption or who are the subject of a special guardianship order. We were not able within the scope of this book to cover the full range of support needs that birth families may have.
- The assessment of support needs for adopted adults (e.g. in relation to searching for members of their birth family) are referred to but are not addressed fully in this book.

The book is intended for all professionals and other staff involved in carrying out assessments of needs for support services. It includes guidance about understanding and assessing the support needs of the children and families involved and describes the services, support and interventions which could assist in responding to the needs identified.

This guidance aims to support the implementation of the Adoption and Children Act 2002 (the 2002 Act) and to provide for the assessment of need for:

- adoption support services as laid out in the Adoption Support Services Regulations 2005 (the 2005 Regulations) and the Adoption and Children Act 2002 Guidance (Children's Services Guidance)

- special guardianship support services as laid out in the Special Guardianship Regulations 2005 and accompanying guidance.

This book uses the DoH et al. (2000b) *Framework for the Assessment of Children in Need and their Families* (the *Assessment Framework*) as its model. As such it looks at the adoptive child and adoptive family's needs holistically, and then considers appropriate support in relation to those needs. Therefore, as well as considering the need for the adoption and special guardianship support services that are described in the Regulations, the book also looks at the need for support services more generally. This means the assessment being carried out, for example if an adoptive family returns to an agency asking for adoption support, is effectively a new Child In Need assessment for the adoptive family (which includes a specific assessment of the need for adoption and special guardianship support services).

The support needs identified in the broad assessment carried out may best be met by an adoption support service, or instead by another service or services, or a combination of the two. The important point is that the identified needs are met with an appropriate coordinated response. Therefore implications may arise for the involvement of a wider range of children's services available within an area, including those provided outside of social services by, for example, schools and primary care trusts. This means that close working between social services and other statutory agencies will be essential when assessments are being carried out and support plans put together.

The requirement to carry out an assessment of needs for an eligible person for adoption support services is a statutory one under the 2002 Act and the 2005 Regulations. The statutory guidance accompanying the 2005 Regulations stipulates that the *Assessment Framework* is to be used as the model when making assessments of support needs. The *Assessment Framework* is issued under section 7 of the Local Authority Social Services Act 1970, which requires local authorities in their social services functions to act under the general guidance of the secretary of state. If there are concerns about the safety of a child which arises during an assessment, as with all other assessments of children and families, workers would need to refer to *Working Together to Safeguard Children: A guide to inter-agency working to safeguard and promote the welfare of children* (DoH et al. 2006).

This book is intended for use alongside the Department for Education and Skills (DfES) *Practice Guidance* (DfES 2005b, 2006) on assessing the support needs of adoptive families and on assessing adopters and the *Assessment Framework* and accompanying *Practice Guidance* (DoH et al. 2000b; DoH 2000a respectively) when considering needs in an adoption or special guardianship context.

How to use the book

Assessment of needs for support services will be carried out by a range of workers, some of whom will have knowledge and experience of the adoption and special guardianship context and others who will not. The book is structured so that it can be used to meet the different needs of staff within this range. It is intended as a resource and the different chapters may be useful at different stages by a range of professionals involved with adopted children and their families.

Chapter 1: The children

- Looks at the characteristics and profile of the children placed for adoption and special guardianship.

- Summarises key themes regarding understanding the needs, concerns and difficulties of children and families involved in adoption and special guardianship and assessing their support needs.

This chapter provides a useful orientation to the context of assessing needs for adoption support services, particularly for workers who are not familiar with adoption and special guardianship. Experienced workers can use the chapter as a reminderof key information and themes.

Chapter 2: The legal and policy context and when to assess

- Describes when an assessment of support needs must be provided, where they should be recorded, who should conduct them and what they should contain.

- Describes the support services which local authorities are required to provide.

- Outlines the role of the adoption support services adviser (ASSA).

Workers can use this chapter when they need to know the stages at which assessments have to be made, by whom, what they should contain and where they should be recorded.

They should consult the chapter if they need information about the support services which a local authority has to provide and how the ASSA may be used as a resource.

Chapter 3: Using the Assessment Framework model

- Outlines key principles in using the *Assessment Framework* in the adoption and special guardianship context.

- Discusses the use of standardised approaches to assessment.

- Explains how to use the *Assessment Framework* at the different points at which assessments of support needs are made, both before and after placement.

This chapter can be used by all workers, as a guide to using the *Assessment Framework* in assessments of support needs. Workers with little experience in using the *Assessment Framework* should familiarise themselves with this chapter.

Chapter 4: understanding the needs

- Looks in detail at understanding the needs of children and families involved in adoption and special guardianship under the key themes of:
  - adoption as a developmental lifespan process
  - the impact of maltreatment and inadequate parenting
  - attachment and loss in adoption and special guardianship
  - identity in adoption and special guardianship
  - challenges in parenting children who are adopted or cared for by special guardians
  - contact with a child's birth family
  - developing 'adoption-aware' services.

Before assessing needs it is important to understand them. This chapter is designed as a reader to help workers gain an understanding of the specific needs of children and families involved in adoption and special guardianship.

Workers who do not have extensive experience in field of adoption and special guardianship can use this chapter on understanding needs in conjunction with Chapters 5, 6 and 7 on assessing needs to inform their assessments. More experienced workers can use the chapter as a resource when they need more information or references about specific themes or issues.

Chapter 5: Assessing adopted children's developmental needs

- Provides guidance for assessing an adopted child's developmental needs.

- Includes guidance on the approach to assessing each dimension and suggestions about the assessment tools that can be used.

- Pointers for practice for each dimension summarise information on understanding and assessing needs and highlight possible support needs.

- Case examples illustrate specific points.

These next three chapters are useful for all workers to guide and focus assessments of need in each of the dimensions of the three *Assessment Framework* domains. The chapters are best used in conjunction with Chapter 4, where a more detailed understanding of needs is required, and with Chapter 8 to assist in analysing the information collected about needs and identifying appropriate forms of support.

Chapter 6: Assessing adoptive parenting capacity

- Provides guidance for assessing strengths and difficulties in the adoptive parenting capacity of adopters or special guardians and identifying whether they may need support.

- Includes guidance on the approach to assessing each dimension and suggestions about the assessment tools that can be used.

- Pointers for practice for each dimension summarise information on understanding and assessing needs and highlight possible support needs.

- Case examples illustrate specific points.

Chapter 7: Assessing family and environmental factors

- Provides guidance for assessing family and environmental factors which may be having an impact on an adoptive family.

- Includes guidance on the approach to assessing each dimension and suggestions about the assessment tools that can be used.

- Pointers for practice for each dimension summarise information on understanding and assessing needs and highlight possible support needs.

- Case examples illustrate specific points.

Chapter 8: Responding to the needs

- Describes how to analyse the information collected to form an assessment of the child and family's needs on which to baseplans for support.

- Outlines different types of interventions and considers providing support related to a range of common needs, difficulties and concerns encountered by children and families:
  - practical and financial support and requests for information
  - settling in and creating a new family
  - the development of an adoptive identity
  - parenting children with emotional and behavioural problems
  - contact with birth families.

- Case examples illustrate support packages developed in response to specific needs or difficulties. Models of adoption support illustrate a range of agency and inter-agency initiatives.

This chapter can be used to guide workers in analysing information gathered and making an assessment of the child and family's needs as a basis for identifying the support/ interventions that would help.

The chapter is also a resource for workers in helping to identify appropriate specific forms of support or interventions for the children and families concerned.

Annex 1

- Annex 1 (pp. 147–160) contains a chart which details the information that can be obtained through the use of the range of evidence-based assessment tools discussed in the book.

Chapter 1

The children

Characteristics of children placed for adoption and their families

The profile of children who are being adopted has changed over recent years; children are now increasingly adopted at an older age, often with some form of contact with members of their birth family (Rushton 2003b; Scott and Lindsey 2003). They are likely to have been looked after within the care system, undergone several moves of placement once they have left their birth family and may have established close ties with foster carers whom they have to leave to join their adoptive family. The ethnic and cultural backgrounds of children being adopted is now much more diverse, and black and minority ethnic children may not be placed with a family of a similar background.

Nearly half (47 per cent) of children between 0 and 17 years old placed from the looked after system for adoption have mental health difficulties, developmental delay, special needs arising from a physical or learning disability or an identified health condition (McCarthy et al. 2003; Meltzer et al. 2000). Most have experienced care that has been inadequate to meet their needs, often from an early age, and many have experienced abuse or neglect or other traumatic experiences (Cleaver et al. 1999). Black and minority ethnic children are likely to have particular needs relating to their racial and cultural heritage and identity (Harris 2003). Children who have been with carers from a different racial or cultural background in earlier placements, or in their permanent placement are likely to have extra support needs, as will with the families who care for them.

Over 15 per cent of adoptions are by foster carers who become the adoptive parents of children they have fostered from the care system (Argent 2003b) these placements have a comparatively high success rate. In view of the history of their relationship with the children they adopt, these foster carers need to understand their shifting role, help the children to understand adoption and negotiate the change of status with the child's birth family where relevant (Ivaldi 2000; Lowe and Murch 2002). Issues related to contact and relationships with a child's birth family may change because of the previous relationship, which may have included a plan for rehabilitation which has not been successful.

Foster carers already have a relationship with the local authority, which also changes when they become adoptive parents. They will already, in partnership with the local authority, be meeting specific needs of the child placed with them, and this needs to be carried forward into the adoption. This will be different from the situation for adoptive parents who are new to the child and birth family.

Birth parents or other birth relatives will often have significant difficulties of their own, which may include psychiatric problems, drug or alcohol misuse or a pattern of domestic violence in the family home. The impact of these difficulties will be reflected in the developmental needs of the child, and may have implications for contact arrangements.

Table 1.1 gives a profile of adopted children in England in 2003.

Potential profile of special guardians and the children they care for

Special guardianship is intended to meet the needs of children for whom adoption is not appropriate, but who cannot return to their birth parents and could benefit from the permanence provided by a legally secure arrangement with their carer. For example, some older children (who may, for instance, be looked after in long-term foster placements) do not wish to be adopted and have their legal relationship with their parents severed, but could benefit from greater security and permanence.

For detailed information on the new special guardianship arrangement, readers should refer to the accompanying *Guidance to the Special Guardianship Regulations 2005*. The information below is a summary only.

Adoption may also not be the best option for some children being cared for on a permanent basis by members of their wider family. Some ethnic minority communities have religious or cultural difficulties with adoption in the form provided for in England and Wales (Rashid 2000), and may wish to use special guardianship, especially given the higher proportion of black children living in kinship care arrangements (Broad 2001). Special guardianship may also be a helpful option for the increasing numbers of refugee or asylum seeking children who are in desperate need of care and permanence but who may have strong ties with their birth families.

Special guardianship is a welcome route to providing a greater degree of permanence for a group of children and young people with complex needs who are being cared for outside their immediate birth family. It recognises that the children and families involved will need support.

Special guardians are likely come from a range of carers, including members of a child's wider birth family, for example grandparents and foster carers. Many special guardians may be caring for children who have ongoing significant relationships and contact with their birth parents. The children are likely to be older than many adopted children, and they may have been in the looked after system for some time. They may present with behaviour that is challenging or have significant levels of physical or learning impairments, emotional disturbance or psychiatric disorder. The children may have been emotionally abused or neglected in the past and have associated attachment difficulties.

Foster carers may differ from others who become special guardians because they will have already worked alongside other professionals, and will have a relationship with the child, knowledge of the child's history and an understanding of the role of the local authority and the child's social worker in the child's life. They also have experience of the child's needs and services already being provided to meet them (Broad and Skinner 2005; Ward 2004).

Table 1.1 Profile of adopted children in England for the year ending 31 March 2003

Looked after children
- 60,800 children were in the care of local authorities on 31 March 2003
- 24,600 children started to be looked after during the year ending 31 March 2002
- 25,100 children ceased to be looked after during the year ending 31 March 2002

Gender
- 55 per cent of children looked after on 31 March 2003 were boys and 45 per cent were girls

Age
- 4 per cent of children looked after on 31 March 2003 were under 1 year old
- 15 per cent were aged between 1 and 4 years old
- 22 per cent were aged between 5 and 9 years old
- 43 per cent were aged between 10 and 15 years old
- 16 per cent were aged 16 and over

Ethnicity
- 81 per cent of children looked after on 31 March 2003 were white and 19 per cent were from black and minority ethnic backgrounds

Placements
- 10 per cent of children looked after on 31 March 2003 were living in children's homes
- 10 per cent were living with their parents
- 6 per cent were placed for adoption
- 68 per cent were living with foster carers
- 7 per cent were in other placements such as residential schools, lodgings and other residential settings

Unaccompanied asylum seeking children
- 2,480 unaccompanied asylum seeking children were looked after on 31 March 2003
- 76.6 per cent were boys and 23.4 per cent were girls

Adoption
- 5,680 adoption orders were made in England and Wales during 2002
- 3,500 children were adopted from care during the year ending 31 March 2003
- 540 children were adopted by their foster carers during the year ending 31 March 2003

Gender
- 53 per cent of children adopted during the year ending 31 March 2003 were boys and 47 per cent were girls

Age
- 7 per cent of children adopted during the year ending 31 March 2003 were under 1 year old
- 59 per cent were aged between 1 and 4 years old
- 29 per cent were aged between 5 and 9 years old
- 5 per cent were aged between 10 and 15 years old
- 0 per cent were aged 16 and over
- The average age at adoption was 4 years 3 months

Duration
For children adopted during the year ending 31 March 2003:
- The average time between entry into care and adoption was 2 years 9 months
- The average time between the best interest decision and adoption was 1 year 8 months

Adoption Search and Reunion: The Adoption Contact Register for England and Wales
At 30 June 2001, there were 19,683 adoptees and 8,492 relatives on the Adoption Register for England and Wales, and 539 successful matches have been made since the start of the Adoption Register in 1991.

Source: DfES 2003b, 2003c.

The children cared for by special guardians are likely to have many similarities with adopted children, though there may be differences, for example in relation to identity issues and contact.

Terminology in this book

We have used the term *support services* to cover collectively both the adoption and special guardianship services as described in the Regulations and wider children and family support services, as unless otherwise stated. When we refer to *support needs* and *support services*, this relates to needs and services that could apply equally to adoptive families and special guardianship families. Where a distinction is necessary between these two permanence options, it will be highlighted. Adopted children and children cared for by special guardians are generally referred to as *adopted children*, adoptive parents and special guardians are referred to as *adoptive parents*, except again where it is necessary to be more specific because of special issues relating to each group. While special guardians and adoptive parents are both undertaking the parenting task in a caregiving or parenting role, it is appreciated that many children cared for by special guardians may not either call or view their special guardians as their 'parents'. References to birth relatives are always clearly identified.

The book uses the term *adoptive family* to describe the family environment in which the adopted child is being brought up. This is intended to cover the wide range of family arrangements which may be involved when children live with a single parent, two parent families, families with or without birth children and families who live in a wider family group.

Key themes in adoption and special guardianship – a summary

Caring for children as adoptive parents or special guardians differs from bringing up birth children in important respects and assessments should take full account of these differences. Some key themes to keep in mind are discussed in detail in Chapters 5, 6 and 7. They are summarised here:

- *Valuing adoptive parents:* Adopters and special guardians should be valued and respected as fulfilling an important role in providing acceptance, good parenting and a lifelong commitment for children with high levels of need and should be approached as partners in assessing support needs.
- *A developmental and lifespan approach to adoption:* Adoption is for life can be viewed as a developmental and lifespan process for all parties in the adoption triangle – adopted children, adoptive families and birth families. Assessments should take into account the stage that the adoption process has reached and the implications for support that may help those concerned.
- *Support needs of children, birth families and adoptive families:* Taking a holistic view of the support needs of all members of the adoption triangle (the adopted child, their birth family and their adoptive family) is likely to promote the welfare and wellbeing of the child.

- *The impact of stressful past events and relationships in the birth family context:* The heritage, experiences and memories that an adopted child imports into their adoptive family has a significant impact on the adoptive family. A child may bring happy memories of times they have enjoyed in their birth families and warm relationships which have been important to them, for example with kind grandparents, or in their foster families. The developmental needs of many adopted children are also affected by earlier experiences of inadequate parenting, including abuse and neglect, domestic violence and other traumatic events. This can result in physical and psychological health problems which tend persist over many years and well into the child's life with the adoptive family (DoH 2002b).

- *Attachment:* All adopted children have experienced separations and loss, which affects their development. Early experiences of separations and loss and adverse relationships with significant parents/caregivers and inadequate caregiving can seriously affect children's capacity to become attached and relate to others. Some may continue to have significant difficulties all their lives.

- *Loss:* Loss is a theme common to all members of the 'adoption triangle'. Birth family members often have a profound sense of loss. Adopted children experience a range of losses and many adoptive families have experienced losses, including those associated with infertility.

- *The child's identity and heritage:* A major task for adopted children is to develop a sense of their identity which incorporates their history with their birth family, including their racial, linguistic, spiritual and cultural heritage. The experience of being adopted on identity and on genealogical continuity needs to be considered when assessing support needs (Owusu-Bempah and Howitt 1997).

- *Challenges in parenting adopted children:* Parenting adopted children has rewards and considerable challenges when adopted children have high levels of need as a result of earlier adverse experiences. Adoptive parents need additional or enhanced parenting skills, and support at times, to be able to respond to the additional needs of adopted children. Interventions may range from information or advice, practical help, training, contact with other adoptive parents, specialist therapeutic help or a multi-agency support package.

- *Contact with the child's birth family:* Continuity and contact with birth relatives can be of great value to adopted children (Macaskill 2002; Neil 2002). Contact can also present significant difficulties for children and adoptive parents and birth relatives. Support may be required to ensure contact arrangements are in the best interests of the adopted child.

- *Developing 'adoption aware' services:* Adopted children have contact with a wide range of services including health, education and social services and professionals in those services should be 'adoption aware', i.e. have an understanding of adoption and its impact on the support adopted children and families need.

Chapter 2

The legal and policy context and when to assess

The legal context

The Adoption and Children Act 2002 (the 2002 Act) requires each local authority to maintain an adoption service, which must include arrangements for the provision of support services. Section 4 of the Act contains the specific duties and powers to assess and provide adoption support, but most of the detail can be found in the Adoption Support Services Regulations 2005 and Chapter 9 of the Adoption Guidance 2005.

The 2002 Act's regime for adoption support was implemented in two phases, the first of which came into force late in 2003. The 2005 Regulations implement the second and final phase. The provisions of the 2003 Regulations are now incorporated into the 2005 version, so there is now no need to consult the 2003 version. The Regulations and Guidance now provide the framework within which adoption support under the 2002 Act has been implemented. All staff working for the purpose of the local authority adoption service on adoption support issues are now covered by the regulations and national minimum standards relating to fitness of staff.

It is also necessary to consider the Adoption Agencies Regulations 2005, which provide the general framework for operation of adoption services under the 2002 Act. The Adoption Agencies Regulations require agencies to address adoption support needs at several key stages in the processes planning, approval, matching and placement. These duties are considered below.

The 2002 Act also creates a regime for the provision of support services to families affected by special guardianship orders. Section 115 of the 2002 Act amends the Children Act 1989 to provide the legal framework for special guardianship. Sections 14A–F of the Children Act 1989 (as inserted by the 2002 Act) provide for the making of, and support services for, special guardianship orders (the power to make special guardianship orders was introduced by the Adoption and Children Act 2002, but was then incorporated into the Children Act 1989, so special guardianship orders are made under the 1989 Act, not the 2002 Act). The Special Guardianship Regulations 2005 require local authorities arrange for the provision of assessments of support need and for special guardianship support services. The *Assessment Framework* is used as the model for assessing special guardianship support needs. Special guardianship is seen as a means of providing children with permanence, so the children cared for by special guardians typically have many needs in common with adopted children. It will therefore come as no surprise to find that special guardianship support assessments and services are almost identical to adoption support services.

When must an assessment of support needs be provided?

There are two kinds of situation where the agency is required to consider adoption support issues. In some circumstances, the agency has a duty proactively to consider adoption support issues, whereas in others, the agency may be asked to carry out an assessment. These are referred to below as 'proactive' and 'responsive' duties respectively.

These trigger points for assessments are discussed in more detail later on in this chapter.

Adopted adults and their adoptive parents have the right to an assessment of their adoption support service needs. These will be assessed by a different assessment route and are not covered in this book.

A birth relative of the adoptive child (other than their birth parents), former guardian or person with whom the adoptive child has an important relationship can request an assessment only in respect of supporting contact arrangements. They are not entitled to an assessment in relation to other adoption support needs.

Similarly, birth parents also have the right to an assessment of their adoption support service needs but this is not covered in this book, except in relation to contact arrangements.

Under the current legislation, no one has an automatic right to adoption support services. Some individuals are entitled to an assessment but in every case the local authority has a discretion as to whether or not to provide services. Based on an assessment, a local authority decides whether to provide services and if so, what services it will provide and in what way. There is no automatic entitlement to services, but an authority must act reasonably in making a decision. In particular, it is important that the authority has clear eligibility criteria and those criteria are applied consistently.

Adoption support services

The 2002 Act (section 2(6)(b)), the Adoption Support Services Regulations 2005 (reg 3) and Guidance introduce a minimum set of adoption support services which local authorities must make arrangements to provide, so that these can be made available to people affected by adoption as the authority sees fit. They are as follows:

- counselling, advice and information
- financial support
- support groups for adopted children and birth and adoptive families
- assistance with contact arrangements between adopted children and their birth relatives
- therapeutic services for adopted children
- services to ensure the continuance of adoptive relationships, including training to help meet special needs of the child and short breaks

'Proactive' duties: points at which the legislation says that the local authority must consider the need for adoption support services

- For the child, when an Adoption Panel is asked to recommend whether a child should be placed for adoption, prior to the agency decision.

- For prospective adopters, when their suitability is being assessed.

- For the child, when information on him or her is shown to prospective adopters.

- For the prospective adoptive family, when a match has been identified between a prospective adopter and a particular looked after child and the Adoption Panel is asked to recommend the placement, prior to the agency decision. This also includes proposals on how the support needs of the prospective adoptive family will be met.

- For the prospective adoptive family, when they comment on the proposed Placement Plan.

- When the placement for adoption of a looked after child is reviewed.

Important: there are no equivalent proactive duties to assess support needs in the context of a special guardianship arrangement and no requirement to place the case before a panel.

Where assessments are recorded

- Recorded in the Adoption Plan, which has evolved from the Care Plan (Guidance Ch 2 para 8).
- Recorded in the Child's Permanence Report to the Adoption Panel.

- Recorded in the Adoption Placement Report, which includes proposals on how the child's needs will be met.

- Recorded in the Adoption Placement Report and then the adoption support component of the proposed Placement Plan, should the placement be approved.

- Recorded in the Placement Plan adoption support component (Adoption Agencies Regs, reg 35 and Sch 5 para 6).

- Recorded in the adoption support component of the Placement Plan.

Note: the Child's Permanence Report, Adoption Placement Report and Placement Plan are discussed in detail in the guidance accompanying the Adoption Agencies Regulations 2005.

'Responsive' assessments: assessments of need for adoption support services that must be carried out by local authorities when requested by

- children who are adopted
- birth children of adoptive parents
- birth siblings of adopted children
- relatives of adopted children
- children who may be adopted
- persons wishing to adopt a child and their existing birth or adoptive children
- birth parents and former guardians of children who have been or may be adopted.

Note: In the case of a special guardianship order, the following people may request an assessment (those marked * are *automatically entitled* to an assessment on request, the others are not, but the authority must consider whether to assess):

- a child (who was previously looked after) subject to a special guardianship order*
- a special guardian or prospective special guardian of a child who was previously looked after*
- a parent of a child (who was previously looked after) who is subject to a special guardianship order*
- other children subject to special guardianship
- other special guardians
- parents of other children subject to special guardianship
- a child of a special guardian – this includes adopted children and children of the family
- a person whom the local authority considers has a significant and ongoing relationship with a child who is subject to a special guardianship order
- a child (not looked after) who is subject to an application for a special guardianship order – this includes a child who is the subject of, or is named in, a local authority report for the court
- a prospective special guardian for a child who is not looked after – this includes individuals who have made an application for a special guardianship order and individuals a court considers should be made a special guardian.

Where assessments are recorded

- Recorded in the Adoption Support Plan (Adoption Support Services Regs, reg 16).

- Recorded in the Special Guardianship Support Plan (Special Guardianship Regs, 2005, reg 14).

- advice, counselling and information
- services to assist where a disruption has occurred or is in danger of occurring
- an adoption support services adviser (ASSA) to help those affected by adoption to access support services.

Clearly local authorities and other statutory agencies such as Primary Care Trusts have a duty to consider the needs of all people in their area, and to provide services ('mainstream services') as appropriate. People affected by adoption will often require, and meet the eligibility criteria for, such mainstream services. This book and assessment process addresses or covers all available services, including both the adoption support services which local authorities are required to make arrangements for and the mainstream services that may also be available to the family from other agencies.

The Integrated Children's System

All assessments of the child should be recorded on the Integrated Children's System (ICS) or Electronic Social Care Record, which, as records are held electronically, allows for the easy transfer of relevant information between different records on the child and his or her care history, including previous assessments of need (DoH 2000b). This is a 'living' system which facilitates an ongoing gathering together and development of information on the child.

Proactive assessments: assessments of needs for support services prior to the adoption order

The Care Plan

A Care Plan is drawn up for any child accommodated by the local authority (Arrangement for Placement of Children Regulations (1991) reg 3). The Care Plan sets out details of the proposed placement for the child and of the management and support of the placement by the local authority. The child's developmental needs are identified and a detailed plan for how those needs will be met is set out, including the support and services to be provided. The Care Plan is prepared by the child's social worker in consultation with other relevant agencies and the child and parents or family members. The child or young person's wishes are taken into account and they are consulted wherever appropriate.

Where adoption is being considered, advice should be sought from the ASSA when appropriate about the plan for adoption, assessing adoption support needs and the provision of support services.

Adoption Plan

When an agency is considering whether a child or young person should be placed for adoption, the child's social worker should prepare an Adoption Plan. As with the Care Plan, the Adoption Plan builds on prior assessments of the child's developmental needs by a range of agencies, for example, drawing on the Initial and

Core Assessments, the Care Plan (which includes the personal educational plan and the health plan), any assessment or statement of special educational need and so forth. The child's Adoption Plan should be reviewed regularly, as part of the normal reviews of the child's case, until a match is identified. The assessment of adoption support needs should be taken into account during preparation of the adoption plan and whenever it is reviewed. This will ensure that information relating to support needs is available and can in due course be incorporated into the Child's Permanence Report and Adoption Placement Report For the Adoption Placement Report, the information should also include proposals on how the child's needs will be responded to (if they are not already being met). Where relevant, advice from the ASSA should be sought.

The assessment of the prospective adopters

The family placement worker will undertake the assessment of prospective adopters. The assessment of suitability has a number of stages – the giving of information, counselling, preparation, checks and references and the Home Study. The assessment process takes in information about the prospective adopters from a range of agencies and sources (for example, Criminal Records Bureau (CRB) checks, medical information, personal references) and this should ensure that the agency has a clear and comprehensive of their potential support needs.

The information collected through these processes is analysed and evaluated and eventually will be put together into a report with an accompanying recommendation to the agency's Adoption Panel that the prospective adopters are or are not suitable to be approved to adopt. The panel's recommendation will then be considered by the agency decision maker, who will decide whether the applicants are approved as prospective adopters.

The worker undertaking the assessment will have in mind throughout the assessment process, the sorts of children who require adoptive homes, the needs those children may have and the qualities and capacities that will be required by adopters who wish to parent them. The approval will however not be limited to a given number, age or gender of children.

The Home Study of the prospective adopters has a structure that is based on the relevant domains of the *Assessment Framework* and so collects information principally in relation to their parenting capacity and their wider family and environmental factors. In considering these domains in relation to prospective adopters, the worker will be identifying potential needs that they may have for adoption support services in general and this information will form part of the report to the Adoption Panel.

The Adoption Placement Report

When adopters have been approved and linked with a particular child, then the worker for the family and the worker for the child should look together at the (already) identified needs of the child, the capacities of the adopters, the general support needs of the adopters and then identify, in addition, what extra and specific support services the adopters will need now and may need in the future to meet the needs of that child.

This information forms part of the Adoption Placement Report. The report therefore includes both an assessment of the needs of all members of the prospective adoptive family *and* proposals as to how those needs will be responded to.

The Adoption Placement Report is prepared by the relevant social worker and then goes to the Adoption Panel for consideration, prior to the agency decision being made. Once the Adoption Panel has made a recommendation about the proposed match, the agency decision maker decides whether to accept the panel's recommendations or not.

This is the key proactive assessment stage for support needs, and use of this book is essential in order to look holistically at the needs of the child to be adopted and the prospective adoptive parents within the new family environment and how these should be responded to. In effect a new Core Assessment from an adoption perspective is being carried out for the prospective adoptive child and their prospective adoptive family, looking in the widest sense at their needs and appropriate interventions (including the need for adoption support services). The ASSA should be consulted during this process. Wherever possible staff from other statutory agencies should be involved in the assessment, as they would be in any other *Assessment Framework* assessment, particularly where there are implications for services that they provide. If such implications become apparent, legislation (Adoption Support Services Regs 2005, reg 14(4)) requires the social worker carrying out the assessment to consult with the statutory agency in question.

The Adoption Agencies Regulations 2005 (reg 32) requires the Adoption Panel to consider adoption support issues whenever it considers a proposed match and empowers it to give advice to the agency. The views of the panel on adoption support needs and service provision will be very useful. They should be conveyed to the agency decision maker and accommodated within the proposed adoption support package so that they are available person(s) whose support needs are being assessed.

The Placement Plan

Once a potential match has been approved, a Placement Plan must be prepared by the family placement worker (or their equivalent) and the child's social worker, with the involvement of the ASSA as necessary. The contents of the Placement Plan are prescribed by Adoption Agencies Regulations 2005 (reg 35(2) and Schedule 5) and include proposals for meeting the predicted support needs of the child and the adoptive family, including details of the support services to be provided. The Placement Plan is finalised once the prospective adopters have agreed its content. Once it has been agreed, the Placement Plan, including its adoption support component, must be reviewed regularly until such time as an adoption order is made or the child has been removed from the prospective adopters. (Adoption Agencies Regulations 2005, reg 36).

The adoption support component of the Placement Plan

Alongside the assessment of need the adoption support component must set out how it is proposed these needs will be responded to. The plan should spell out clearly the

- objectives and the key services to be provided
- time-scales for achieving objectives
- individual worker who will be responsible for coordinating and monitoring delivery of the services
- respective roles of others responsible for delivering services
- criteria that will be used to evaluate success
- procedures that will be put in place to review the services to be provided and the objectives, including the timing of reviews.

After the adoption order is made, the adoption support component of the Placement Plan continues in its own right as an Adoption Support Plan under the Adoption Support Services Regulations 2005 (reg 16).

Reviews

Under the new Placement Plan review arrangements, within each review there must be a consideration of support needs and how they are being met. The Adoption Agency Regulations 2005 (reg 36(6)(b, c, e, f) state the following must be considered as part of the review:

- the child's needs, welfare and development, and whether any changes need to be made to meet his or her needs or assist his or her development
- the existing arrangements for contact, and whether they should continue or be altered
- the existing arrangements for the provision of adoption support services for the adoptive family and whether there should be any reassessment of the need for those services
- in consultation with the appropriate agencies, the arrangements for meeting the child's health care and educational needs.

A full reassessment of support needs will be required only if there have been significant changes in the circumstances of the child and adoptive family.

The local authority must review the provision of support services if any changes in the person's circumstances come to their notice, routinely at regular intervals and whenever a specific timetabled course of action within a plan comes to an end

Responsive assessments: assessments of needs for support services from an eligible person

This refers to any assessment carried out at the request of any of the persons who are entitled to request an assessment and are most likely to occur after (perhaps many years after) an adoption order has been made. An adoption support team may deal with these requests where local authorities have such a team in place, or alternatively, they may be responded to by a referral and assessment team. It is important however that, if the request is dealt with by such a generic team, the members of the team and their managers are 'adoption aware' and understand in particular how adoption support differs from family support in other contexts.

Stage 1 – Initial Assessment

When a request is received that relates to an adopted child or the adopted family in the context of the adopted child, an Initial Assessment using the *Assessment Framework* should be carried out to identify the needs of the adoptive family in question, including, but not limited to, the need for adoption support services. The worker carrying out this assessment should refer to this book in order to (re)familiarise themselves with adoption-related needs and support interventions, in conjunction with guidance on the *Assessment Framework* (DoH et al. 2000b: paras 3.8, 3.9, 3.11). The Initial Assessment may identify support needs, including needs for a specific adoption support service, and propose an appropriate response.

Stage 2 – Core Assessment

If more complex issues arise and it is decided a more in-depth assessment is required to ascertain the support needs of the adopted child or adoptive family, a Core Assessment will be undertaken using the *Assessment Framework*. When carrying out this assessment, workers should use this book in conjunction with the *Assessment Framework Practice Guidance* (DoH 2000). The advice of an ASSA may, as usual, be sought regarding the assessment of adoption-specific needs and the identification of support services and interventions.

- When a Core Assessment of this nature is being carried out and the adoption context emerges as a key factor, workers are effectively conducting a similar exercise to the proactive assessment undertaken at the matching and placement stage for children being placed for adoption.
- The initial and core assessments should identify and seek to build upon the strengths of the adoptive family, but occasionally some adoptive families experience such severe difficulties that it is necessary for the local authority to take action, possibly including statutory intervention, to safeguard the welfare of the adopted child. Workers must keep this possibility in mind and, if appropriate, initiate inquiries under section 47 of the Children Act 1989.

Circumstances where a full assessment is not required

Where a request for assessment relates to a particular support service, or it appears that the person's needs may be effectively responded to by a particular support service, a brief initial assessment may be all that is necessary (Adoption Support Services Regulations 2005, reg 13(2)).

Certain forms of information and counselling described in the 2002 Act are not included in the adoption support service 'provision of information, advice and counselling' definition. These include

- the provision of birth records information under section 60 and associated counselling under section 63 of the 2002 Act
- counselling on the adoption process and ramifications of adoption for birth parents, children and prospective adopters under regulations 13, 14 and 21 of the Adoption Agencies Regulations 2005.

Note however that intermediary services under the Adoption Information and Inter-mediary Services (Pre-Commencement Adoptions) Regulations 2005 *are* adoption support services (reg 3(3)).

There are also some adoption support services that an authority would be expected to provide to everyone without need for any assessment; for example responding to requests for general information. Persons affected by adoption also of course have the right to access public services like any other individual through the usual channels.

Assessing the need for financial support

As already outlined, the 2002 Act gives people affected by adoption the right to request an assessment for their adoption support needs including financial support. The Adoption Support Services Regulations 2005 give local authorities the power to pay financial support to adoptive families. Regulation 8 describes the conditions that need to be met for an adoptive family to be eligible for financial support, and Regulation 15 outlines how authorities should arrive at the amount to be paid. Regulation 9 contains important restrictions on the payment of remuneration to former foster carers who go on to adopt.

It is important to remember that there is only one system of adoption support, of which financial support is a part, and financial support needs should not be consid-ered in isolation from other needs. Adopters may approach the agency requesting financial support only, but workers should *as a minimum* consider whether to carry out a wider assessment, even if the adopters are convinced that money is the only kind of help they need!

Proactive assessments

For proactive assessments of prospective adoptive families carried out using this book we expect that consideration of financial assistance should be an implicit and automatic part of the assessment process. This includes looking at one-off payments to facilitate the placement and whether the adoptive family requires regular ongoing financial payments to help cover the costs of the upkeep of the adoptive child. It will be particularly important to address financial issues at an early stage where a child is to be adopted by existing foster carers, as the loss of basic and enhanced fostering allowances may represent a severe blow to the household economy and be a source of severe anxiety.

Responsive assessments

Eligible persons have the right to request an assessment of their needs for adop-tion support service, including the need for financial support. In responsive assessments consideration of financial support is to be made as the worker making the assessment deems appropriate, given the nature of the need being expressed by the person(s) who have requested the assessment. However, it may be apparent following the Initial and/or Core Assessments that the support need in question relates to, for example, a CAMHS intervention rather than a difficulty in managing financially due to the upkeep of the adoptive child; and therefore consideration of the need for financial support is not necessary.

If a request is made by an eligible person that relates *specifically* to an assessment of their financial support needs (as opposed to their support needs generally) an assessment of needs for financial support has to be made, but a wider assessment of need should at least be considered.

Using the Assessment Framework in a financial support context

As the worker undertaking the assessment works through the assessment process, he or she should continually be thinking of any implications for financial expenditure. Certain dimensions within this guidance will have particular relevance in this regard, for example (this list is not exhaustive).

Dimension(s)	Possible related expenditure
Health; Emotional and Behavioural Development; Self-Care Skills; Basic Care; Stimulation	Item costs associated with special or additional needs
Housing	Costs of extensions or even moving house. Adaptations for disabled children.
Wider Family	Costs of travel to facilitate contact arrangements.

Workers undertaking assessments may find it most helpful to look at all the financial implications for someone being assessed within the Income dimension of the Family and Environmental Factors Domain in Chapter 7. Crucially, it is in this dimension that the basic upkeep costs of the adoptive child should be considered, and it will be useful to look at these alongside other expenditures that have been identified. These can then be compared to the means of the family in order to decide if financial support is needed. See Chapter 7 for more detail.

When working through the 'Providing information, practical support and financial support' section of Chapter 8, the recommendations for financial payments that have been arrived at following consideration in Chapter 7 should be recorded.

What happens following the assessment

It is important to keep in mind that, while there is in certain circumstances a duty to carry out an assessment of need for adoption support, the agency does not owe a specific duty to provide adoption support services following an assessment. Even where an assessment identifies a need for support, the agency still has a discretion as to whether or not to provide the service. This makes it important to manage the expectations of families during the assessment stage.

Where there has been a 'proactive' assessment of support needs as part of the adoption process, the assessment will form part of the Adoption Placement Report which will then be considered by the Adoption Panel, who may give advice to the agency.

Following a 'responsive' assessment carried out at the request of an eligible person, the responsible worker will agree the outcomes of the Initial or Core Assessment with colleagues (including those from other statutory agencies). The worker will then pass their findings and recommendations on to their manager, who will make a decision in the light of the agency's procedures and eligibility criteria.

Then, under Regulation 17 of the Adoption Support Services Regulations 2005, the local authority is then required to produce a proposal of what adoption support services will be provided. This should wherever possible include also any proposals relating to service provision by other statutory agencies. Notice of this proposal must be given to the adopters whose adoptive child/family has been assessed. In proactive cases this proposal and notice will take the form of a draft Placement Plan which adopters may make representations about.

Following this period in which the adoptive family may make representations, the local authority is required (Regulation 18) to make a formal decision as to whether the person(s) assessed have a need for adoption or special guardianship support services and if so whether any services will be provided.

If services are to be provided, a support plan is then drawn up in accordance with Regulation 16 and its associated statutory guidance. For proactive cases, this will be the adoption support component of the Placement Plan. Again, all services that are to be provided from any statutory agency should be included in this plan if possible. The practitioner who carried out the assessment of needs should be involved in this process.

The adoption services support adviser

The responsibilities of the adoption support services adviser

Each adoption agency is required (Adoption Support Services Regulations 2005 reg 6) to have a single point of contact on adoption support, an ASSA who can signpost people affected by adoption to appropriate services, give advice and information and encourage the accessing of relevant services and benefits. (There is no equivalent requirement in relation to special guardianship support.)

The ASSA is required to have a good knowledge in the following areas, and be able to act as a consultant and resource for colleagues:

- the adoption context generally
- the adoption process and the impact on all concerned
- the agency's legal responsibilities in relation to adoption support
- the relevant DfES *Practice Guidance* and its use
- the use of the *Assessment Framework* in the assessment of needs for support services
- appropriate forms of support and intervention for adopted children and their families

- local services who may be involved in providing support, including social services, health, education, housing and leisure services and voluntary and specialist agencies.

The ASSA also has a role in:

- advising the agency in relation to assessment, support services and support plans
- ensuring that suitable intra- and inter-agency arrangements are in place between local social services, education, local health trusts, other local authorities and voluntary agencies where they are involved; the voluntary sector often has an important role to play in contributing to an assessment and providing services to a family in the context of adoption and special guardianship
- assisting colleagues to facilitate the involvement of relevant agencies and services in the assessment process
- acting as an advocate for individual families where necessary, to influence the provision of services for families across agencies and to ensure that issues and concerns are fed back into the local children and families strategic planning process
- ensuring the early involvement of relevant agencies who either are already involved in delivering support to the child and/or family, or where their services may be required, dependent on the needs of the assessed person(s); staff from relevant agencies need to be involved at an early stage so that the assessment is carried out with the benefit of their professional expertise and so that they can provide advice about appropriate interventions and support.

The role of the adoption support services adviser

The role of the ASSA carries a range of responsibilities. These responsibilities will not all be performed by the ASSA personally; many will be allocated to different staff within the agency.

Chapter 3

Using the *Assessment Framework* model

The *Assessment Framework*

The *Assessment Framework* provides a systematic way of analysing, understanding and recording what is happening with children and young people within their families and the wider context within which they live (Figure 3.1). It focuses on three interrelated systems or domains: the child's developmental needs, the capacity of the parents to respond to the child's needs and the impact of any family or environmental factors on the child's needs or the parenting capacity.

Many children in the adoption and special guardianship context are children in need of support and the *Assessment Framework* should, therefore, be used when assessing their needs and those of their family members.

The *Assessment Framework* (DoH et al. 2000b) and accompanying *Assessing Children in Need and their Families: Practice Guidance* (DoH 2000) provide advice and guidance about conducting assessments with children in need and their families and should be referred to in conjunction with the DfES *Practice Guidance* on assessing adopters and on the support needs of adoptive families, as well as this book.

Principles of assessment and the *Assessment Framework*

The *Assessment Framework* sets out the core principles underpinning effective assessments of children in need and their families (DoH et al. 2000b: p. 10 para 1.33). These also apply to the assessment of adoption support needs. Assessments should

- be child centred
- be rooted in child development
- be ecological in their approach
- ensure equality of opportunity
- involve working with children and families
- build on strengths as well as identify difficulties
- be a continuing process, not a single event
- be carried out in parallel with other action and providing services
- be grounded in evidence-based knowledge.

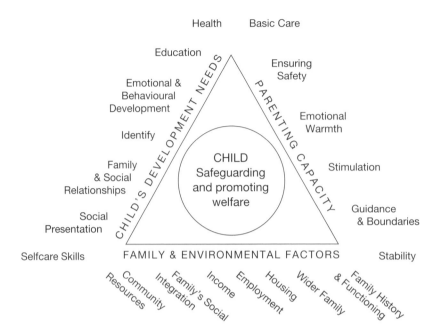

Figure 3.1 The *Assessment Framework*.

Applying these principles to assessing needs for adoption support services

Application of these principles is important when assessing support needs. This includes

- giving adopted children a voice
- developing collaborative working partnerships with adoptive families and with relevant members of the child's birth family
- taking account of the views of the adopted child and adoptive family
- considering the impact of diversity and discrimination at all stages of the assessment process – this is ensuring equality of opportunity
- using approaches to assessment that engage and have relevance for all family members
- using a range of approaches, including evidence-based approaches, rather than relying on one approach to ensure the quality and reliability of assessments
- take an inter-agency approach to assessment and provision of services.

Each of these will be explained more fully in the following paragraphs.

Giving children a voice

It is essential that children have a voice in the assessment process as appropriate to their age and understanding. Workers need to use approaches to communicating with children in a manner that encourages and enables children to participate in the assessment process (Jones 2003). Staff working with adopted disabled children and their families always need to remember the importance of inclusion and of using age appropriate and adapted approaches for communicating with disabled children (Stalker and Connors 2003). Staff working with children who have had early adverse childhood experiences, including maltreatment and loss, need to take a child developmental approach which also takes into account the impact of such adverse experiences when helping children and young people to communicate and to take part in the process of planning for their current and future needs (Cooper 2005; Rustin 2005; Schofield 2005).

Developing collaborative working partnerships with adoptive families

Assessment approaches to assessing adoption support needs should always focus on identifying and building on strengths in the adoptive family which enable them to respond to the needs of the adopted child. Assessment should also take into account the unique and specific impact caring for a child with high levels of need can have on family life. Adopted children's difficulties can continue or emerge for many years after placement despite being placed in a well-functioning family.

Adoptive families have been through a lengthy assessment process before approval and may be apprehensive about a further assessment process. Adoptive parents are chosen for their strengths, resourcefulness and resilience and they may have a clear idea of the support they would like or they may have concerns that they wish to explore further. They may have been trying to deal with challenges relating to caring for their adopted child for some time and blame themselves, or expect others to blame them, for not being able to resolve difficulties they may have. They need to be related to as central players in finding a possible solution to the difficulties being encountered rather than the cause of the problem (Archer 2000a, 2000b, Archer and Gordon 2005).

Workers therefore need to build a supportive working partnership with the adoptive parents and work with them to find out together what their child's and their own support needs are and to plan a support package. It is usually helpful to start working with the adoptive parents by focusing both on their current concerns and the areas in which they feel they are doing well. The assessment can then move forward to assess the current needs of the child and adoptive parents, and any relevant family or environmental factors, and identifying the interventions or support which would help to respond to those needs.

Working with birth families

An assessment of an adoptive child's support needs will often involve working with the birth family and the child, and workers should seek to develop as positive and supportive a relationship as possible with the birth family so that those concerned can work together in the best interests of the child. This may involve working collaboratively with the independent social worker for the birth relatives. The issue of ongoing contact between the child and the birth parents (and how this might be supported) will be one of the key considerations in many assessments of support needs.

The views of the adopted child and adoptive family

It is essential to keep the views of the adopted child and family members central in the assessment and planning process. Adoption support is valuable only if it relates to what the adopted child and adoptive family want and can use. It is easy to assume that particular needs should be prioritised or that certain interventions would be helpful without having asked the individuals concerned what they would like to happen and in what sequence.

Considering the impact of discrimination and diversity

The diversity of patterns of family life and the role of friendship groups and of supportive birth family members and other people who are significant to the child need to be understood. The uptake of adoption support services by black and minority ethnic adoptive and birth families is lower than might be expected and agencies should ensure that support services are accessible and appropriate for this group of children and families (Charlton et al. 2005; Harris 2005). Assessment approaches should also seek to understand the adopted child or child cared for by special guardians within the context of their previous families they have lived in and of the impact of any adverse circumstances, including disadvantage and discrimination on both the child and family.

Using approaches to assessment that engage and have relevance for all family members

The *Assessment Framework* focuses on identifying strengths as well as any difficulties. A balanced, evidence-based assessment – one that recognises resilience, resources and protective factors in adoptive families and birth families, as well as addressing needs or difficulties – forms a sound basis for developing effective strategies for providing support and resources.

Taking an inter-agency approach

Children who are adopted or cared for by special guardians are often involved with a range of agencies. It is important to ensure that assessments of support needs are contributed to by the relevant services concerned with children and families and involved the development, delivery and review of support plans. Education and health services are often central in supporting the specific needs of adopted children and their early involvement in the assessment of support needs where relevant is crucial. Where required, workers may need to ensure that such services take an 'adoption-aware' approach taking into account the specific needs of chid which relate to their being adopted.

The use of the *Assessment Framework* in assessing adoption support needs

The *Assessment Framework* provides the conceptual map for structuring assessments of children in need and their families in a variety of circumstances. Effective planning is based on good assessments and revisiting the *Assessment Framework* is useful to remind workers of aspects of the child and family's life, which may need to be considered when assessing support needs.

In the adoption context we have to remember the importance of the child's experience in their birth family, and how the child's experience in their birth family, the heritage and sense of identity they bring with them to adoption and the meaning and impact of any continuing contact. Conceptually we need to bear in mind the relationship between two families for the child and therefore for some of challenges (and rewards) the adoptive family may be encountering. The *Assessment Framework* triangle in the adoption context may therefore be represented as illustrated in Figure 3.2.

The child's developmental needs are central to any assessment of needs for support services. The adoptive family provides the core environment for promoting the development and welfare of the child. The task therefore is to assess the needs of the child and what support services the child and their adoptive family, and members of the birth family where relevant, may require in order to respond to the child's identified developmental needs.

All prior assessments of the child, the child's birth family, of the child while in earlier placements and of the prospective adopters should have been based on the *Assessment Framework*. The Integrated Children's System (ICS) provides the framework gathering, recording and analysing for all work with children and families, and planning interventions and identifying outcomes those interventions are intended to achieve (DoH 2000b). The assessment of needs for support services should take into account that the adopted child is a member of the adoptive family and has the heritage of having been born into their birth family. The past and current involvement of members of the birth family in the child's life and their impact on the child has to be incorporated into an assessment of needs for adoption support services.

Using standardised evidence-based approaches to assessment

There are a range of approaches to making assessments of support needs and it is helpful to use a combination of approaches when making an assessment. This book recommends the use of evidence-based approaches as part of the process of the

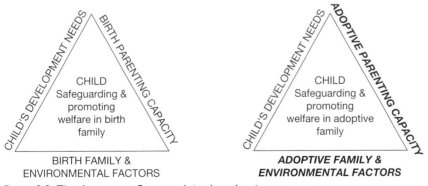

Figure 3.2 The *Assessment Framework* in the adoption context.

assessment of adoption support needs, so that assessments are based on clear and systematic ways of collecting and analysing information. Standardised approaches using assessment tools which are grounded in good practice and empirically validated help to provide results that can be well evidenced, i.e. the evidence on which professional judgements are based can be clearly communicated.

Using standardised tools allows the comparison of needs across different contexts – for example, comparing the child's needs in their birth family, when with substitute carers, their likely needs when joining an adoptive family and their needs once in placement.

The assessment tools produced to support workers using the *Assessment Framework* provide a range of standardised evidence-based approaches to interviewing children and families and assessing their needs. They are helpful as a resource pack or tool kit in assessing support needs and can be used in various combinations and alongside other assessment approaches already is use, including where agencies have developed their own tools for undertaking assessments.

The HOME Inventory

The Home Observation and Measurement of the Environment (*HOME*) *Inventory* is a standardised way of interviewing a parent or main caregiver with the key child in the home by systematically talking through a typical day for the child in detail (Cox and Walker 2002; Joyce 2003). It focuses on exploring and assessing the nature and variety of a child's day-to-day experiences, the quality of the child's home environment and the parenting capacity of the caregivers from a perspective that is as close as possible to that of the child. The *HOME Inventory* allows the worker to explore key issues about the child's care needs, parental responsiveness to the child and relationships with other family members. It helps to develop a profile of the child's needs within the context of adoption or special guardianship, and to predict the level of support required to assist the family to respond to the child's needs.

The Family Pack of Questionnaires and Scales

An interview using the *HOME Inventory* can be added to by using relevant questionnaires and scales from the *Family Pack of Questionnaires and Scales* (DoH et al. 2000a) to explore particular individual and family issues, such as parenting hassles, family activities and aspects of individual health and wellbeing. Like the *HOME Inventory*, the *Questionnaires and Scales* are particularly useful for opening up discussion with family members and can be used to provide an indication of possible areas of need or difficulty where support may be necessary.

The Family Assessment

The *Family Assessment* provides a flexible approach to understanding children within the family context, which may be used with birth families, substitute carers and with adoptive families and special guardians and their families (Bentovim and Bingley Miller 2001). The *Family Assessment* facilitates the exploration of key areas of family relationships and family life including family organisation (roles and responsibilities, problem solving, decision making, managing conflict and relationships with the wider family and community) and parenting (providing stimulation, nature of attachments and guidance, care and management of the children), as well as how family members communicate, how feelings are dealt with, the nature of key relationships in the family and how identity issues are handled.

The family history component of the *Family Assessment* allows for the exploration of the impact of the past experiences of individual family members in their current life. This might be, for example, to help understand the impact of a child's past history on their current developmental needs, or how past significant events experienced by adoptive parents (e.g. infertility) may be affecting how they relate to their child. It is useful in more complex family situations where an assessment of adoption support needs is required.

The Attachment Style Interview for Adoption and Fostering

The *Attachment Style Interview for Adoption and Fostering* enables the practitioner to assess the attachment style of adopters and foster carers and the support systems in terms of their partner and very close others in whom they can confide and how they use their support systems, particularly at times of stress (Bifulco et al. 2002a, 2002b). This is helpful when assessing adopters and also to identify their potential adoption support needs and how they can best be delivered.

The In My Shoes interview

In My Shoes is a computer-assisted interview for communicating with children and vulnerable adults (Calam et al. 2000). The programme is designed so that a trained adult sits alongside the child and assists, guides and interacts with the child through a structured interview process. The practitioner works with the child through a series of modules which are designed to help the child to share information on their experiences and emotions with different people in home, educational and other settings. The *In My Shoes* interview has proved effective for a range of purposes which include:

- enabling a child to talk about their experiences, thoughts, feelings and wishes
- helping a child to talk about their experience of living in their current, or previous family or other care settings
- gathering a child's wishes and feelings about being fostered, moving to an adoptive family
- talking about school with a child – learning, friendships, relationships with teachers and others.

It therefore has obvious value in the adoption field in assisting practitioners to communicate with children at different stages of the adoption process about a range of aspects of the adoption experience.

Ways in which these assessment tools can assist in making assessments of adoption support needs are indicated throughout the book. Workers require training to support their use in practice and to apply them effectively in the adoption and special guardianship context. Annex 1 (pp. 147–160) contains a chart which details the information that can be obtained through the use of the range of evidence-based assessment tools discussed in the book.

The process of making an assessment: using the *Assessment Framework* at the different stages when assessments of support needs are made

The model for making an assessment using the *Assessment Framework* is useful when assessing support needs. The model involves a process of assessment, analysis and planning which has a number of stages, as follows:

- Collecting information about the needs in each of the dimensions in each domain, i.e. adopted child's developmental needs, parenting capacity and family and environmental factors.
- Analysing the relationship between the dimensions of each domain, e.g. how the different needs of the adopted child affect each other.
- Analysing the interrelationship between the dimensions of the different domains, e.g. how the strengths and any difficulties in the parenting capacity of the adoptive parents are contributing to the child's developmental needs being met or not met, and the impact of any relevant family and environmental factors on either the child's needs or the capacity of the parents to respond to those needs. The assessment should also identify any concerns about a child's safety.
- Using this analysis to identify the support needs of the adopted child and family. It may also include any support needs of the child's birth family or others who have been significant to the child.
- Deciding what support, interventions and services will be most effective to respond to the identified needs of the child and family and establishing the outcomes that would indicate the interventions had been successful.

The worker's first task, therefore, is to collect information about each of the dimensions in the three domains of the child's developmental needs, parenting capacity and family and environmental factors so that they can gain an understanding of the child's current developmental state within the context of their family and environment. As discussed, standardised approaches to assessment can be used as part of the process of collecting relevant information and evaluating needs.

Chapters 5, 6 and 7 describe how to assess a child's developmental needs, adoptive parenting capacity and family and environmental factors, looking in detail at each dimension of each domain. Chapter 8 considers in more detail how to draw together and analyse the information collected and make the assessment of the needs of the adopted child and family, which forms the basis for identifying the support required, and looks at different forms of support.

Using the Assessment Framework at the different points when assessments of support needs are made

The process for using the *Assessment Framework* to assist in assessing the needs of adopted children and families and the interventions or support to help respond to those needs differs according to the stage at which the assessment is being made.

Assessing support needs at the Care Plan and Adoption Plan stage

The process for assessing a child's support needs is similar whether at the Care Plan or the Adoption Plan stage. Building on prior assessments, the child's developmental needs should be reviewed and ongoing support needs of the child identified, e.g. specific health care needs, ongoing therapy for emotional difficulties, or access to groups or activities related to the child's religious or cultural needs. Any specific parenting skills and/or experience likely to be required to respond to the needs of the child (i.e. parenting capacity) should be identified. A child's strengths and areas of resilience should always be noted alongside their needs to provide a balanced assessment.

This information can help to predict what support future adoptive parents may potentially require to support them in caring effectively for the child, e.g. information and advice about managing a child's medical condition, help with liaison with schools, advice about accessing relevant services. Family and environmental factors which may affect either the child's developmental needs or the parenting capacity of future adoptive parents should be noted and potential support needs identified. These may include financial assistance, support with contact for the adoptive or birth family, or access to community resources.

The assessment of adopters

Practice Guidance has been issued by the Department for Education and Skills (2006) to guide the assessment of adopters. The preparation and assessment of prospective adoptive parents includes an assessment of their potential support needs. These support needs will be identified in the context of assessing the prospective adopters' capacity to parent children with the profile of needs generally associated with adopted children. They may therefore require, for example, further training or contact with other adopters to learn more about particular aspects of adoption. Potential support needs related to the assessment of family and environmental factors may arise, e.g. in relation to financial assistance, housing adaptations or planning support with contact with the birth family.

Foster carers who become special guardians will have been through an assessment to become foster carers and therefore information relevant to their support needs as special guardians will be available. They are likely to be well attuned to the assessment process and, in general, alert to their support needs. They will however require support to help them to take over the exercise of parental responsibility and to manage working relationships and contact arrangements with the child's birth parents and family, tasks which will previously have been undertaken by local authority. When family members from a child's immediate or wider family apply to become special guardians, they may require/benefit from careful encouragement to consider support needs.

The Placement Plan

The preparation of the Placement Plan involves a bringing together of information from the previous assessments, including the assessment of the support needs of adopted child and the adoptive family as described in the Adoption Agencies Regulations 2005 and their accompanying guidance. The adoption support component of the Placement Plan is based on a careful and thorough review of the identified support needs of the child and family in the context of the planned match, to ascertain whether any additional support is needed either by the child or the family. This involves reviewing the child's developmental needs, as set out in the current Care or Adoption Plan, in the light of the specific match and the prospective adopters' capacity to meet the needs of the particular child. Identifying the strengths and resilience of adopted children and adoptive parents, which balance out their needs, forms an important part of the assessment. Again the impact of any family and environmental factors specific to the match which may affect the child's developmental needs or the adoptive parents capacity to care for the child should be considered.

This process enables the worker to identify the specific support needs of the child and family (including birth relatives where relevant) and plan an effective support package. The adoption support component of the Placement Plan should also predict potential future support needs and identify routes for having those needs assessed. A support package for a child with physical impairments and a learning disability and his or her family, for example, might include the arrangement of ongoing support by a special teaching assistant for the child in school, access to training for adoptive parents in managing the child's troubling behaviours, access to short breaks once the child has settled, advice and consultation about contact with birth relatives, financial assistance for the birth parents in attending contact and financial assistance to adapt the adoptive family house to suit the needs of the child. White adopters who are going to adopt a child from a minority ethnic background may require support in building links with people or groups from their child's community.

Responsive assessments: requests for assessments of needs for support services after an adoption order has been made

Once an adoption order has been made, the need for support can arise in many different ways and at different points in the child or young person's or their adoptive family's development. Adoptive parents are chosen for their qualities of resilience, resourcefulness and the ability to act as advocates for their children and it should not be treated as a sign of failure that they return to the agency to ask for help. It is also important to remember that sometimes the need may be identified by the adopted child themselves or a birth child in the family. It will take some courage on the part of the child to make contact with formal services and agencies should ensure that they have appropriate arrangements in place to support young people who come directly to them. The same is often true for birth relatives, who may also request an assessment.

Whoever it is that asks for help, the person they turn to will depend on what the problem is, whom they feel they can trust and who is most appropriate. So for instance, where there is a health problem, they will usually go directly to their general practitioner (GP) or other health professional; where there are difficulties at school, they will talk to the teacher. Others may be talked over with spiritual advisers or community leaders or friends. Sometimes this may result in a referral to the local authority for an assessment of adoption support needs but in most cases, people will get the help they need from the person they first requested it from.

Many adoptive families approaching social services for assistance will already have prior assessments and adoption support plans in place that should inform any assessment under the Adoption and Children Act 2002. This will not be the case for non-agency adoptions and for parents who adopted some years ago, though there will be information from the time the adoption order was made.

Adopted children, their adoptive parents and other family members may ask for help in a variety of different ways. They may come with a request for information or advice, for example, which can be provided without further assessment. They may have a clear idea of what the problem is and come with a request for further services, or they may come with concerns and worries but not be clear about the exact nature of the problem and where it is located. Birth family members may also seek support, for example with maintaining contact. Social workers will need to call on their skills in creating the conditions which enable people to talk openly about how they see the problem now, how it has developed over time, who experiences it most acutely and what potential solutions might be. It is essential that workers undertaking assessments are 'adoption aware' and understand the potential impact on adoptive families of caring for a troubled or traumatised adopted child, and that adoptive parents do not feel blamed for the difficulties they are encountering.

Children and young people may need to be seen separately, as may their adoptive parents. It is important to remember that different members of the family may have different perspectives on the problem, how it affects them and what potential solutions may be. Social workers will need to give constructive feedback on how they understand what has been said as well as their own perspective. This should not only focus on problems but also give recognition to the strengths of individuals or the family as a whole and the desire they have to change or improve. Where the problem seems to involve many factors or be of significant complexity, a specialist assessment may be required. On rare occasions, there may be safeguarding issues involved when a child's safety and wellbeing within the adoptive family will need to be assessed.

Initial and Core Assessments

The principles underpinning making an Initial Assessment or a Core Assessment are similar. Both involve an exploration of the current concerns, and how they relate to, first, the child's developmental needs, second, current areas of strengths and difficulty encountered by the adoptive parents in caring for the adopted child, and third, any relevant family and environmental factors. This forms the basis of assessing the support needs of the child and family. The difference between Initial and Core Assessments is in the depth of the assessment undertaken.

When an Initial Assessment is undertaken in response to a request for an assessment concerning a particular problem, the worker should check round the *Assessment Framework* triangle domains and dimensions to make sure they have all information they need to decide how to proceed. It may then be apparent what support or service is required to respond to the problem. Alternatively, the assessor may feel they need more in-depth information before recommending a particular service or form of support, in which case they will move onto a core assessment. When using the *Assessment Framework* for a Core Assessment, the assessor may focus on certain dimensions more than others in the light of the findings of the initial assessment. The definitions of Initial and Core Assessments as used in the *Framework* will apply in this guidance (DoH et al. 2000b).

The range of concerns prompting a child or family member to make a request for support may be adoption related or may be related to difficulties common to other children and families rather than being adoption specific. The worker undertaking the assessment should ascertain whether the child's needs or the concerns expressed by the child or family are adoption related or not adoption related to determine whether this affects the appropriate response, seeking the advice of the ASSA when necessary.

Chapter 4

Understanding the needs

Key themes

Adoption as a developmental lifespan process

Adoption is a lifespan developmental process that has different tasks at different stages for each member of the family.

For the adopted child these stages include the following:

- *Pre-adoption*
- The period when the child is with their birth family.
- The period when decisions are being made about permanency, where the child is likely to be placed in a foster family; this may include a period of 'twin-track' planning, when reunification and permanence are being considered simultaneously.
- The development of plans for contact with the birth family and others.
- Matching a child or young person with a permanent family who can respond to the child's needs.
- The process of placement and early settling of the child.

- *Adoption*
- The making of the adoption or special guardianship order (which is often especially significant for older children).

- *Post-adoption*
- The longer-term development of the relationships between the child and their new family.
- The managing of ongoing contact with the birth family and/or previous carers in the child's best interests.
- The transition to independence for adopted young people and the adopted child becoming an adult.
- Being an adopted adult, which itself has a series of developmental stages.

The adoptive family have developmental tasks alongside those of the adopted child outlined in the adoptive family life cycle (Table 4.1: adapted from Scott and Lindsey 2003). Workers and many adoptive parents may find them useful in the context of assessing support needs.

Table 4.1 Adoptive family life cycle

Stage	Adoptive parents' tasks	Adopted children's tasks
Pre-adoption	Coping, where relevant, with loss, e.g. infertility and not being able to be a biological parent. Helping own parents and siblings, and children (if any) accept plan to adopt.	For older children, trying to cope with loss of birth parents, and uncertainty about future.
	Coping with prolonged evaluative assessments, and anxiety of not knowing when they may be offered a child.	Coping with difficulty of knowing they will lose current foster parents.
	Preparing for social stigma of adopting.	Coping with anxiety about future adoptive parents.
	Preparing for life-style change, e.g. giving up job, change in relationship with partner.	
	Coping with feelings about accepting a child who may not be 'ideal'.	
Infancy	Taking on the identity of adoptive parents and finding acceptable role models.	Relinquishing past attachments with birth parents and others.
	Developing realistic expectations.	Developing primary attachments to new caregivers and secondary attachments with key members of wider adoptive family.
	Integrating them into the family.	
	Persisting with affection and establishing secure attachment even if faced by personal disappointment.	
	Exploring thoughts and feelings about birth family.	

Stage	Adopters' tasks	Adopted person's tasks
Preschool	Beginning the telling process.	Learning elements of adoption story.
	Creating an atmosphere conducive to openness about adoption and talking about birth family.	Questioning adoptive parents about adoption.
Middle childhood	Helping child accept the meaning of adoption, including loss of birth parents, possible anger (especially directed towards adoptive mother).	Coping with the losses related to being adopted.
	Helping child develop a positive view of birth family.	Exploring feelings about being given up by birth parents, developing an acceptable story around being adopted.
	Managing any contact or communication from birth family.	Coping with stigma of sometimes encountered relating to being adopted.
	Coping with insecurity that telling may engender; worrying child may want to leave or not love adopters.	Validating dual connection to both families.
Adolescence	Helping young person develop own sense of identity including recognition that traits may come form birth family; accepting difference from some of their values and style.	Integrating adoption into a secure sense of identity.
	Supporting search interest and plans, and helping to develop realistic expectations.	Exploring feelings about search process. Finding balance between idealisation and vilification of birth parents.
	Coping with adolescent rebelliousness with a sense of proportion, coping with feelings that young person may wish to leave home as soon as possible thus rejecting the love they gave.	Trying to understand extent to which feelings and behaviour are typical for adolescence and which may derive from being adopted.

Birth families and a lifespan approach

Birth families go through a sequence of stages, according to the circumstances of their child's adoption, which workers need to consider as part of their assessment of support needs whether ongoing contact is planned or not. This includes all the steps leading up to the plan for their child to be adopted, which may involve assessments concluding they are not able to provide the care their child needs. Birth parents have the experience of losing their child to adoption, whether or not they agreed with the plan. Beyond that they live with the enduring loss of their child and having to deal with contact, lack of contact and/or reunion if it occurs.

CHILDREN'S DEVELOPMENTAL NEEDS

The impact of maltreatment and inadequate parenting

Children joining adoptive families or special guardians import a set of memories, expectations and ways of relating which are based on their experiences in their birth families and later substitute families. These experiences may include separation, loss, abuse and neglect and other trauma. An understanding of the impact of these experiences on their emotional and behavioural development is central to assessing the support they may require.

Health

An adopted child's medical history begins before birth and pre-birth traumas can include exposure to violence (including attempted abortion), maternal rejection, maternal illness, poor nutrition and the use of alcohol, tobacco and drugs (Mather 2003).

The potential effect of parental misuse of substances such as alcohol, drugs or tobacco, in pregnancy, which can affect the developing brain of the unborn child (McNamara 1995), is an example of the close relationship between child's health and development and parental physical and mental health. Parental alcohol misuse can lead to Foetal Alcohol Syndrome or Foetal Alcohol Effects Syndrome, which is often undiagnosed but potentially just as debilitating. Long-lasting negative effects on the child include learning difficulties, low intelligence quotient (IQ), poor socialisation skills, poor coordination, memory problems and brief attention span.

Inadequate parenting, including abuse and neglect, domestic violence, and other traumatic experiences, have an impact on a child's physical and psychological health and the difficulties tend to be persistent over many years (DoH 2002a; Cleaver et al. 1999; Glaser 2000). Looked after children have high levels of diagnosable mental health disorders and the likelihood of a child having more than one condition is high. Problems may include attention deficit disorder, conduct disorders, depression and attachment difficulties (Quinton and Rutter 1988).

The degree of their difficulties is associated with their age at placement (Quinton et al. 1998; Sellick et al. 2004) and the severity of their experiences of abuse, neglect or attachment problems and how early they encountered these difficulties (Bentovim 2006; Howe 1998). Adverse experiences that occur at a preverbal stage of development can have a particularly damaging effect on a child's emotional development (Glaser 2006).

Education

Adopted children may have learning problems or difficulties at school related to their earlier experiences of trauma, abuse, neglect or separations and loss. It has been demonstrated that trauma in the first ten years of life is likely to impair a child's brain and body function, emotional health and cognitive functioning (Cairns 2001; Glaser 2000). There may be language and memory problems, lack of coordination, numbness (insensitivity to pain and discomfort) and psychosomatic illness. Traumatised children may be in a permanent state of arousal that leads to inattention, or display behaviour that is disruptive.

There is an increased risk of exclusion for some adopted children who underachieve at school due to a lack of skills in developing and sustaining relationships and for those who develop oppositional behaviour. Exclusion can then lead into associated problems, such as drug and alcohol abuse, involvement in criminal activities, teenage pregnancy and, for a few, suicide attempts. The effects can be cumulative for children who have experienced a range of abuses, so that, for example, sexually abused children who also have birth parents who are violent, or severe in their parenting, are sometimes more at risk of becoming sexually abusive themselves as they grow older (Bentovim 2002, 2004; Cleaver et al. 1999; Skuse et al. 1998).

The educational and cognitive development of adopted children can also be influenced if previous caregivers were unable to provide the relevant support, e.g. in households where there were chaotic patterns of care so that children had no consistent routines or help with reading or homework.

More is now known about the possibilities for a child 'catching up' on developmental delay following severe early deprivation and this helps to explain the impact of early and serious neglect on children. A large study of young children (most of whom were seriously developmentally delayed and malnourished) adopted into the United Kingdom from Romanian orphanages (Beckett et al. 2003; Farina et al. 2004; Rutter et al. 1998a) were followed up at 6 years of age; Rutter et al. (2001) showed that the majority had caught upon their physical and cognitive development to a remarkable extent. However, a substantial minority had continuing social or behavioural problems that affected their capacity to make secure attachments and to understand and manage the rules for social relationships.

Emotional and behavioural difficulties

Children who are placed beyond infancy may have had experiences of family and social relationships, which were frightening, unresponsive, neglectful, when they were exposed to risk and danger or to a family climate of high levels of conflict and disruption. They may have been socially isolated and have had little support or involvement from their extended families. Adopted children's expectations and their responses to family life and social relationships in their new family may reflect those experiences. They may use their earlier adaptive responses, which are inappropriate in their new setting and can provoke distress or even rejection in the new family.

Adopted children who have grown up in a context of neglect, but who have not been physically or sexually abused, often respond rapidly, in terms of their physical wellbeing, to a context of good care. This response is often noted in foster care, and usually continues in their permanent families. However, adopted children who have been neglected can be the most emotionally damaged and among the most difficult children to care for.

Quinton et al. (1998) found that children adopted between 5 and 9 years old had higher rates of difficulty and underachievement than younger adopted children, increasing as children's age goes up. They found that 48 per cent of the children studied had moderate to severe 'conduct disorders', 49 per cent had emotional problems, 23 per cent were hyperactive, 29 per cent had problems with bed wetting and soiling, and 43 per cent had significant difficulties in their relationships with other children. Intellectual and school performance was significantly lower in this late adopted group.

Factors contributing to the range of emotional and behavioural difficulties adopted children experience

Factors found to contribute to the serious range of difficulties experienced by the children in this and other studies included:

*   serious mental health and other problems of the birth parents
*   the children's experiences of abuse and neglect and inadequate parenting
*   emotional challenges for older children associated with leaving their birth parents and later carers to whom they may have become attached
*   the significant tasks involved in shifting and developing new attachments, establishing a sense of identity and integrating their past life with their new life (Dance and Rushton 2005b; Quinton and Rutter 1988; Rushton and Dance 2004).

Building resilience: supporting emotional and behavioural development

Building resilience is key to recovery from adversity (Gilligan 2000). Resilience comprises a set of qualities that helps a person to withstand many of the negative effects of adversity. Different elements of resilience include self-esteem, self-efficacy, self-reflexivity, social empathy and autonomy (Howe et al. 1999). Resilience is not just a matter of constitutionally inherited strengths. It can be greatly enhanced by the quality of the relationships and the environment in which the child grows up.

In order to develop resilience, children need

*   to have a secure base or safe haven from which to explore
*   to know their story and develop a positive sense of their identity
*   to develop their self-esteem (the sense of how they measure up to their own expectations and those of people close to them)
*   to develop a sense of self-efficacy (believing that one's efforts make a difference).

Resilience can be enhanced by a child feeling connected to key people, in particular their birth and adoptive/foster family. Resilience is promoted by school experiences that are positive and supportive and maximise the child's potential and by positive involvement in leisure activities, team and individual pursuits, volunteering, caring for animals, groups and so on. Adoptive parents, special guardians, ASSAs and all other professionals engaged with the child can work together to promote resilience (Monck 2003).

Attachment in adoption and special guardianship

Attachment is a key concept in the context of adoption and special guardianship. While there are many different views and ongoing research about the application of attachment theory in practice, it is a useful framework for giving us ways of understanding the difficulties many adopted children have in developing trusting and secure attachments with their new caregivers (Prior and Glaser 2006). A network of secure attachments forms the basis for positive emotional and behavioural development and the bedrock of successful family and social relationships. Insecure attachments have a serious impact on a child's emotional and behavioural development and their capacity to form social and family relationships. It is important that workers making assessments of adoption support needs are able to recognise attachment difficulties in children and ensure that children and families have access to the advice and support they require, including appropriate specialist help.

Adopted children who have experienced maltreatment, separation and loss may find it particularly hard to form secure attachments and to demonstrate appropriate feelings and behaviours to new adult caregivers. Recent thinking and research in the field of attachment has resulted in a growth of knowledge that helps us to understand their difficulties.

The development of attachments

Newborn infants are extremely vulnerable and remain so for several years. In order to survive, they must receive care and protection. Attachment theory suggests that they are born with a range of behaviours that are designed to obtain proximity to a caregiver (usually a parent). Known as *attachment behaviours*, they include crying, clinging, following and smiling. Attachment behaviours are activated when the child feels vulnerable or in danger. Their goal is to alert the caregiver to respond to their needs. Appropriate responses produce feelings of safety and wellbeing in the child. When attachment behaviour is not activated, the child is free to explore, play and learn (exploratory behaviour). Exploratory behaviour is suppressed by attachment behaviours (Bowlby 1969), which are concerned with the physical and emotional survival of the child and take priority.

Within their close relationships, young children begin to develop *mental representations* or *internal working models* of their own worthiness, based on the availability of caregiver(s) and their ability and willingness to provide care and protection (Ainsworth et al. 1978). As Howe (2000) suggests:

> Within each care giving relationship, the self will be experienced as more or less loveable, interesting, effective and worthy of care and protection. Similarly, children will experience attachment figures as more or less available, responsive, sensitive, interested and accepting.

Internal working models contain expectations and beliefs about:

- one's own and other people's behaviour
- the lovability, worthiness and acceptability of the self
- the emotional availability and interest of others, and their ability to provide protection.

Patterns of attachment

Based on empirical findings, four combinations of the way the self and others are incorporated into internal working models have been proposed (Howe et al. 1999):

- secure patterns
- ambivalent patterns
- avoidant patterns
- disorganised patterns.

Secure patterns

Children experience their caregivers as available, responsive and protective and themselves as loved and lovable. They have a strong sense of their caregiver as a *secure base* from which they can venture into the world, confident that they can return in times of need. Children with secure attachments have good self-esteem and self-efficacy and learn to deal effectively with feelings of distress, anxiety and anger. The ability to make sense of the self and others in relationships increases social competence.

Ambivalent patterns

Children with ambivalent attachments experience their caregiver as inconsistently available (e.g. children whose birth parents or caregivers misuse drugs or alcohol) and responsive and themselves as dependent and poorly valued. These children may wish to remain close to their caregiver at all times, becoming distressed and clinging at the threat of any separation. This may be combined at other times with attempts to force the caregiver to stay close through coy or coercive behaviour, such as screaming, shouting, being aggressive with the caregivers or brothers and sisters.

Avoidant patterns

Children with avoidant attachments experience their caregivers as consistently rejecting and themselves as compulsively self-reliant. They tend to avoid seeking care when they are distressed or aroused. Instead they behave in a way that is apparently 'self-sufficient' appearing not to need comfort from adults. However, physiological measures such as heart rate and other signs of anxiety show that, despite their lack of care-seeking behaviour, such children are in fact highly physiologically aroused at times when they are likely to be stressed, for example, on separations and reunions (Spangler and Grossman 1993).

Disorganised patterns

Disorganised patterns are often associated with children who have been maltreated by their caregivers: children with disorganised attachments experience their care-givers as either frightening or frightened and themselves as helpless, angry and unworthy of care. For these children, care represents danger and they feel safe when looking after themselves and controlling others. Disturbing behaviours such as reck-lessness, hypervigilance, frozen states and aggression to self, others and animals can develop (Lyons-Ruth 1996). Research suggests these children are likely to have con-flicting representations of the same caregiver behaving in contradictory ways (Steele et al. 2003). Elements of disorganisation are likely to be present in the majority of late-placed adopted children, given the early adversity that most have suffered.

Case example – contradictory internal working models for attachment figures*

The prospective adoptive parents of Steven, a 10-year-old boy, were concerned that the degree of support they had been offered while he was placed with them initially would lessen considerably once he was adopted. They were concerned about extensive masturbatory behaviour that drew attention to him in school. Steven had special needs but with learning support was able to be integrated into a mainstream school. He also showed some worrying sexual interests in younger children.

He had been placed in foster placement and subsequent adoptive placement following removal from his birth family. There was evidence of considerable rejection by his mother that persisted despite a number of attempts to rehabili-tate him to her care. She was able to care more satisfactorily for two younger sisters, which in itself had considerable impact on the boy. He was also seri-ously physically abused and treated cruelly by a stepfather. In a phase of earlier play therapy he revealed extensive sexual abuse in addition to the physically abusive experiences which he recalled. A specialist interview revealed that he continued to be deeply affected by the traumatic aspects of his abuse and remained fearful of being found and abducted by this individual, who he felt would seek revenge because he had spoken about the abuse perpetrated against himself. At the same time, his stepfather, this abusive, frightening figure, had urged him to behave in a similar way to him. In this way he had been a per-mission-giving figure which led to the boy identifying with his aggressor. This is commonly seen in boys subject to extensive abuse and exposed to a climate of violence and abuse of the sort perpetrated against himself and his mother. It became clear that, if this placement were to succeed, an extensive therapeutic package would be required to support both the boy and the adoptive parents set up between the Social Services Department, who will have a continuing con-cern about his wellbeing, as well as the local CAMHS and specialist services for children who have been abused and are at risk of behaving abusively.

* All case examples have been anonymised and have had details changed to ensure confidentiality

The impact of adopted children's early attachment difficulties on later relationships with significant caregivers and others

Each of these patterns of behaviour are adaptive to the caregiving situations that adopted children have experienced in their early months and years of life. They make sense (in that they help the child to deal with feelings of distress and anxiety) in the context of particular relationships and they may become highly developed. Thus, even when children have been severely maltreated, they will show attachment behaviour, albeit of an insecure or disorganised type. Only in unusual situations such as institutions, profound neglect or serial caregiving, will children show weak or no attachment behaviour when they are under stress (Archer and Gordon 2004; Beek and Schofield 2004a; Howe and Fearnley 2003).

There is a link between the pattern of attachment and the way the adopted child regulates his or her emotional life, showing striking internalising or externalising response to frustration, and the child's sense of self. Disorganised patterns are associated with a negative sense of self and difficulty in trusting others (Howe and Fearnley 1999).

Over time and in the same caregiving context, internal working models will tend to stabilise, self-confirming and resistant to change. They developed as adaptive coping responses to particular caregiving patterns. When children are placed in new families where responsive caregiving is readily available, former models cannot be erased but new internal working models develop slowly, 'superimposed' on previous models. These latter may persist and re-emerge under stress. We now know that children who have been traumatised at a young age may continue to live with strong feelings of fearfulness or aggressiveness as a result of the impact of seriously aversive experiences on their neurological development (Glaser 2000; Prior and Glaser 2006).

If there have been elements of fear and helplessness in adopted children's previous relationships with caregivers, they may have learned to keep themselves disengaged from the caregiver. They have come to see caregiving as dangerous and therefore will not allow the carer to occupy the caregiving role. Therefore, caregiving responses that normally help children to feel secure have the effect of heightening their anxiety and they repel the advances of their adopters. Their strategies can be experienced by their adopters as aggressive and controlling. These are the children most commonly diagnosed as having 'attachment disorder'. When faced with such behaviours, it is understandable that adoptive parents begin to feel helpless and sometimes hostile and relationships can feel increasingly out of control, and children and parents may need specialist help with building more secure attachments (Archer and Burnell 2003; Hendry and Vincent 2002; Hughes 2003).

At school, the emotional states of many adopted children impact on their relationships with adults, teachers and peers and potentially disrupt their learning in addition to any specific learning difficulties they may have. Teachers may need briefing on the effects of childhood trauma so that the child is fully understood and their needs can be met appropriately.

Family and social relationships

In their wider family and social relationships, some adopted children with attachment difficulties find it difficult to join in with normal social activities for children of their age. For example, adoptive parents may find their child cannot easily manage at children's clubs or groups or other social activities or after school clubs. They may lack the language, social skills and ability to join in cooperatively with peers that means they are not integrated into the group or are seen as disruptive or 'naughty' by other adults.

Other experiences can affect adopted children's attachments. For example, adopted children from black and minority ethnic groups may have internalised racist attitudes that delay the development of more secure attachments in a black family. Alternatively, for some children, these internalised attitudes may promote particular patterns of attachment in a white family, which can result in their full personal growth being delayed because of the difficulty they have in integrating their racial identity (Prevatt Goldstein and Spencer 2000).

Loss in adoption and special guardianship

Loss is an integral part of adoption for all parties and affects adopted children, birth families and adoptive parents, except perhaps for adoptive parents who have their own birth children. Adopted children have experienced a loss of their relationship with members of their birth family and their capacity to attach to new caregivers can be affected if they are unable to grieve these and associated losses effectively. At various points in their development, different aspects of loss may become more significant and the child and/or family may need help in understanding and managing the child's experience of loss. Brodzinsky et al. (1998) take a developmental or 'family life cycle' perspective on the theme of loss in adoption that can help to identify, understand and respond to a child effectively.

Brodzinsky's (1990) influential 'stress and coping' model of adoption adjustment summarises the nature of loss in adoption in the following five points:

- loss of biological parents
- loss of stability in relationship with adopters
- loss of 'self'
- loss of genealogical continuity
- 'status loss' of feeling different.

It is argued that before the age of 6, young adopted children cannot fully comprehend the meaning of adoption. For those adopted as infants, adoption is simply a 'label', associated with the story that has been conveyed by adoptive parents and accepted without much question. For those placed beyond infancy, there is a similar absence of full understanding of the legal context and irrevocable nature of adoption.

By about 6, children gain a fuller sense of the losses involved in adoption. As greater awareness of family relationships develops, so does a greater awareness of the loss of the biological family. Questions about the reasons for the adoption become more urgent and troubling to the child. Adopted children can acquire a sense of rejection, abandonment and unworthiness. Anxieties about the fragility of birth family relationships can be transferred into the adoptive family. This can give rise to the process of 'adaptive grieving' often apparent in middle childhood and adolescence.

Developing a positive sense of identity in adoption and special guardianship

The development of a positive sense of identity is a key theme for children in this context. Children who are adopted or cared for by special guardians need to develop an appropriate balance in their sense of themselves as a member of their adoptive family as well as having a heritage and connections with their birth family and two cultures and communities.

Children who are permanently separated from their birth families face additional psychological tasks in relation to developing their sense of identity (Triseliotis et al. 1997). These include

- (re)attaching to new adoptive parents
- dealing with the awareness of adoption, which involves not only knowing you are adopted and understanding the meanings and implications of this, but also access to genealogical and other background information
- coping with the notion of two sets of parents and acknowledging the differences involved
- dealing with the sense of loss of the original family and the element of rejection that it conveys
- forming of an identity that includes all these attributes.

Identity development

Identity development therefore encompasses at least two key questions for adopted children. The first is to understand '*Who am I?*' This is essentially about knowing one's own history including the history and characteristics of one's birth family. For adopted children, understanding information about their personal history and birth family is likely to involve incorporating information about difficult events and parental characteristics such as mental illness, substance misuse, abusive behaviour and so on.

Consideration should be given to how adopted children will incorporate this type of information in building their sense of self-esteem. A wholly negative view of birth relatives is unlikely to help adopted children to feel good about themselves. An unrealistically positive view of birth relatives may create difficulties for children in relating to their 'real' adoptive parents, and may led to disappointment if reunion occurs later.

The process of developing a sense of personal history will vary according to the child's age when first separated from the birth family. Adopted children separated at a very young age will have no conscious knowledge or memories of their birth families and so are entirely dependent on other people to convey important information to them. Therefore the potential for fantasy, feeling confused or feeling a significant 'gap' is greater than for the older placed child.

Adopted children who have memories of their birth families may have difficult memories which lead to a confused sense of where they belong and mixed loyalties. But they will, to a certain extent, have some personal knowledge of their history.

The second central question for an adopted child is '*Why was I adopted?*' Not only is this again about knowing one's own history but also it involves questions about the motives of birth parents or relatives in failing to care for child adequately, or relinquishing a child. Children may question their own worth or whether they can be loved. For some adopted children, even those placed as tiny babies, knowledge of their adoption brings about a multifaceted sense of loss and/or rejection.

The needs of children from ethnic minorities

Adopted children from ethnic minorities face potential difficulties in feeling a positive sense of their ethnic identity as a result of experiencing discrimination, marginalisation or the lack of opportunity to mix with people with a similar identity. This may be the case, even when children are in basically stable adoptions with loving and committed parents (Harris 2005; Kirton and Wooger 1999).

In order to develop a positive sense of their identity, adopted black or minority ethnic children need adoptive parents or special guardians who can help them to value their race, ethnicity and culture. Parents who share aspects of the child's cultural/ethnic background are likely to find this task easier. Parents who are from a different background have additional hurdles to overcome in meeting the child's identity needs (Greenwood and Foster undated; Thoburn et al. 2000).

Black minority ethnic children placed with families from a different ethnic and cultural background have a visible sign of their difference as adopted children and so are likely to have to manage how to tell their adoption story earlier than other children may have to. Families who are isolated from the ethnic communities of their children may need support in locating the community networks their children require.

Adopted black and minority ethnic children and families have to cope with managing the 'differences' involved in being adopted or cared for by special guardians as well as the impact of living with racial discrimination and other experiences of discrimination and oppression which can damage their self-esteem and sense of competence and belonging. They and their adoptive and birth families have the right to assessments of their support needs by professionals who recognise the impact of diversity and discrimination on children and their families (Charlton et al. 1998; Harris 2005).

Refugees and unaccompanied asylum seekers often have experienced severe trauma, abandonment, loss and death of relatives, resulting in extra support needs which may require a range of supports.

The needs of disabled children

Adopted children who have a physical or learning impairment, or who have a physical illness have at least two lifelong factors that affect their wellbeing and development – their illness or impairment and adoption. Disabled children have a right to assessments by who understand about both the fields of adoption and disability and to coordinated specialist services that meet their needs (Argent 2003a; Cousins 2006).

Disabled adopted children need extra help to develop a positive sense of identity and to be assured of their rights to life opportunities. They and their families, however, face many barriers in accessing otherwise universally available services or opportunities. Adoptive parents may need support with ensuring that their children can take part in ordinary activities and opportunities that enhance their sense of identity and self-worth, for example, membership of clubs and school activities, going on school trips, going on holidays, taking part in sports or other hobbies (Argent 2003a; DoH 2000).

Self-care skills

Many children who are permanently removed from their birth families have had to become independent in their self-care or to take age-inappropriate responsibility for the care of brothers and sisters. In the same way, some children have had to take up the carer role in relation to their parent(s) because of, for example, parental disability, physical or mental ill health or drug or alcohol abuse. These young carers often continue to carry a burden of guilt, responsibility and acute concern about their parent(s).

Adopted children who have become used to having to be independent and self-sufficient, may reject the care offered by adoptive parents or special guardians. Older adopted children may refuse to allow an adoptive parent to respond to a younger child's needs. These processes frequently become evident during assessment for permanency planning when a sibling group is placed in foster care. The difficulties a child may have in either accepting the care they need, or seeing their brothers or sisters receiving appropriate care, are likely to persist into a permanent placement.

Case example – children who continue to take a protective role

Johnny and Sidney are two boys aged 6 and 4 years who have been placed in foster care following the separation of their birth parents after many years of domestic violence. The boys are very close to one another and Johnny sees his role as protecting his brother. He also worries about his mother. Sidney had a positive relationship with his father and misses him. Their adoptive parents are struggling to parent the children, who have little trust in the adults around them. The boys are also aggressive in their play and Johnny had been excluded from school for stabbing a child with a sharp pencil. Using the *Family Assessment* (Bentovim and Bingley Miller 2001) was revealing and made it easier for the children to speak about aspects of their past rather than their current placement, and for the adoptive parents to understand more about the impact of the children's past experiences. Talking with the adoptive parents themselves with the boys present about family communication helped to develop a discussion with the boys about how families and parents work together. This helped the boys to feel more secure. Further individual therapeutic support was required to help the boys to settle.

Alternatively, other children respond to a context of neglect with dependent responses and become reliant on the care of others. This reflects their immaturity and failure to progress through early stages of self-care.

PARENTING CAPACITY

Challenges in parenting children who are adopted or cared for by special guardians

The adoptive parenting tasks and challenges need to be understood when assessing and planning support and may best be considered using the *Assessment Framework* dimensions of the parenting capacity domain.

Basic care

For some adopted children the quality of basic care received prior to placement has been poor and this may affect both their general health and their response to their new family environment. For others, their previous experiences of abuse may have led them to distrust or reject basic care in their new families.

Some adopted children with attachment difficulties have a desperate need to try to control every aspect of their lives. Parents may find that despite providing good quality basic care, there are in battles over everyday issues, such as dressing, washing, cleaning teeth, food and mealtimes and bedtimes (Archer and Gordon 2004; Hendry and Vincent 2002). This may be due to anxiety, mistrust, poor self-esteem, the need to feel 'in control' or underlying depression. Managing these struggles can be intense, persistent and exhausting and adoptive parents may not have the capacity to provide the care the child needs without support.

Case example – difficulties over basic care

A mother who was concerned about her 4-year-old adopted daughter Rosie, who was exhibiting temper tantrums, refusal to comply with routine matters such as eating, washing and dressing, excessive and compulsive drinking, was referred to a CAMHS team and individual psychotherapy assessment provided for the child with regular consultations with the mother. Very little information had been available about Rosie's birth mother, who abandoned her at a few months' old, but Rosie's work with the psychotherapist had enabled her to explore ideas and fears about mothers in her life and the consultations with the adoptive mother helped her to understand the difficult behaviours in a different way and to begin to reduce the frustrations and tensions in their relationship in the home environment.

Many adopted disabled children require high levels of basic care and will continue to do so indefinitely. Providing such care can become more onerous as children become heavier and sometimes less cooperative and adoptive parents become older.

Ensuring safety

All adopted children need to be kept safe at a level that matches their age and stage of development and capacities. A key task for adoptive parents at the beginning of a placement is to get to know the level of protection their adopted child needs to ensure their safety. They then have to adjust and adapt their care in ways that maintain the child's safety while promoting their developing independence.

Adopted children of various ages can present challenges for adoptive parents in keeping them safe, for example, the tendency of some children with attachment difficulties to be over-trusting of strangers. These may stem from early trauma and attachment-related difficulties, or behaviour learned from a previous caregiving environment or genetic predisposition.

There are a range of behaviours in older children that require adoptive parents to be particularly alert to ensuring safety which include

* impulsivity and risk taking
* aggression and violence
* self-harming and addictive behaviours
* running away
* sexualised behaviours
* indiscriminate affection
* lying and stealing.

The first principle of caring for these troubled children is to manage primary issue of ensuring safety and protection – for themselves, the adoptive family and others who come into contact with them (Archer 2000b).

Parenting an adopted sexually abused child may present particular issues including issues of safety. An adopted child with sexualised behaviours may create sexual feelings, trigger painful memories, and expose vulnerable areas of family life. The experience of being sexually touched by a child can be especially traumatic (Macaskill 1991).

Protection from bullying and harassment is important for all children and may be particularly significant for adopted children who have difficulties in social relationships, are known to have a care history, from black and minority ethnic children and disabled children. Some research indicates that while many white adoptive parents of black adopted children understand about racism in theory they do not always link it with their own adopted child and therefore may fail to understand and protect them (Kirton and Wooger 1999).

Adopted children with learning disabilities may be particularly vulnerable to approaches by strangers who wish to take advantage of their readiness to respond in a trusting way. A study found that adoptive parents of children with Down syndrome were particularly concerned about their children's safety when unattended inside the home and outside the home, due to their natural friendliness and indiscriminate attitudes to strangers (Mason et al. 1999).

Emotional warmth

All adopted children who have experienced separations and losses, including those with attachment difficulties or those who have experienced abuse or neglect, have a particular need for consistent attuned and responsive caregiving from their carers.

All adoptive parents hope that their adopted child will respond to the emotional warmth they provide, and in time emotionally 'claim' their adoptive parents as parents, and the majority find that this is the case. But we know that a significant number of children will take longer to respond and some may always have limitations in this area. Caring for adopted children who are unable to respond to their adoptive parents love and affection can be a painful, frustrating and exhausting experience.

Even in infancy, the traumatised child's defensive strategies may push the caregiver away. In intact mother–infant dyads, it is the caregiver's contribution that will be the most significant in determining the quality of the attachment. A study of fostered infants showed that the fostered infant brings a past that has a significant impact on the relationship (Stovall and Dozier 1998). Even highly sensitive carers may struggle in these conditions.

Caring for troubled adopted children can reveal or reactivate emotional difficulties experienced by adoptive parents and families. Troubled children are hypersensitive to the states of others, and can have a heightened awareness of the vulnerability of their caregivers – this can heighten the vulnerability of both. This makes adoptive parents living with a traumatised child particularly at risk of their own attachment issues being reactivated.

Research by Steele et al. (2003) has given us a way of understanding how traumatised and maltreated children build trusting relationships with their new parents over a period of time. Many of the adoptive mothers in the study had had difficult childhoods but had been able to resolve their feelings about their experiences and move on. They demonstrated resilience, the capacity to be reflective and thoughtful about children's needs and were often particularly compassionate towards the traumatised children in placement, who made good progress. Some mothers however had not been able to 'process' their own unhappy experiences, which therefore remained 'unresolved'. As a result they were unable to focus adequately on the needs of their adopted children or use an organised strategies to deal with some of the conflicts presented by the children, who did not make good progress. Workers therefore need to be sensitive to possible unresolved feelings related to past loss or trauma and ensure that adoptive parents have access to therapeutic help.

Stimulation

Many adopted children have lacked stimulation in their early months and years (this has all been said above in various places). Adoptive parents have to be able to provide stimulation and encouragement and opportunities for communication and play that enable such children to develop their capacity to learn, explore and play and develop their potential.

Cognitive development may be delayed and there may be significant gaps in the adopted child's social development and experience. Adoptive parents may have to learn new skills to be able to provide the stimulation, play and learning opportunities to meet the particular needs of their child and in learning how to communicate in ways that promote their cognitive development.

Guidance and boundaries

All adopted children require guidance and boundaries suitable to their age, stage of development and unique needs, within a framework of support and stability. They can then develop into secure, autonomous, independent and responsible adults.

Providing adoptive parents with appropriate parenting strategies has been the focus of much work in the adoption field (Adoption UK 2000; Archer and Burnell 2003; Gordon 2003). Many adopted children respond well to the provision of clear boundaries and guidance and adoptive parents do not require help in this area. Some require only advice about managing the everyday challenges which setting new boundaries for a child who has joined the family can bring.

Some adopted children affected by early trauma, the regulation of emotions and the development of internal controls are two things they find extremely difficult. This puts enormous pressure on adoptive parents because of the extremes of emotional responses and dysfunctional behaviour which the children present.

Many of the adopted children for whom it is harder to find placements have experienced birth parenting which was marked by high levels of inconsistent care, changing caretakers, inconsistent boundaries, inappropriate levels of punishment or failure to manage behavioural difficulties. Considerable parenting skills are required by adoptive parents to establish and maintain boundaries and manage issues of control and guidance for such children.

Some, though not all, adopted children and young people, who have been exposed to a context of instability, inappropriate disciplinary patterns, punitive or inconsistent care, respond with challenging and oppositional behaviour as an understandable coping strategy. They may tell lies or steal or develop destructive or aggressive behaviour. Adoptive parents often find this challenging or concerning and they may seek support.

If boundaries in the new family are uncertain or inconsistent or guidance is unclear, this can confirm an adopted child's belief that caregivers are unreliable and lead to an increase in their anxiety. Firm boundaries enable a child to feel safe and contained, and are a precursor to change (Archer 2000b).

Stability

Adopted children who have experienced many disruptions in their lives often find managing change more difficult than other children. This includes normal changes such as transition from one year to the next in school, change of child-minder, going away on holiday and can result in the child displaying difficult behaviour which is challenging for adoptive parents to cope with.

Adoptive parents can experience difficulties in feeling emotional warmth for adopted children who are angry, rejecting and resistant to change and this can make it hard for them to respond effectively to their child's emotional needs (Archer 2000a, 2000b; Greenmile 2003). In one study of 5–9-year-old children placed for permanence in middle childhood, 27 per cent of the parents reported that the children had not formed an attachment relationship with one or both parents after the first year. These parents said it was difficult for them to relate to their children in a warm responsive manner and that this problem had increased over the year (Rushton et al. 2003).

Contact with a child's birth family

Purposes of contact

Contact may serve a number of different functions for the adopted child, which vary over time (BAAF 1999). When assessing the support needs related to contact, it is important to have a clear idea of the purpose of the contact, i.e. which particular needs of the child is it intended to meet (Neil 2002; Triseliotis et al. 1997). The quality of contact can then be defined in terms of the extent to which it helps to respond to those needs.

Contact can contribute to meeting an adopted child's needs by

- enabling a child to feel that birth parent(s) are supportive of new family and reducing feelings of guilt in forming close relationships with the adoptive family
- enabling a child to feel thought about or cared for by members of their birth family
- promoting stability by providing continuity and staying in touch with significant people
- reassuring a child about the wellbeing of relatives
- enabling a child to develop realistic understandings of reasons for separation from birth family and to understand that the reasons for separation were not their fault
- enabling a child to grieve loss and reduce feelings of rejection
- providing knowledge and information about family history can help child avoid fantasising about background; maintaining child's connectedness to their community of origin
- maintaining flow of information which could facilitate face-to-face contact later on if it is wished for by the adopted child or person
- letting the child know that the new family accept that they have a range of feelings about their birth family
- helping a child develop a positive and clearer sense of their identity, including clearer self-images and physical identity.

Contact can present difficulties for an adopted child and their adoptive and birth families (Hundlebury 1997), including the following:

- Open adoption is likely to stretch the capacity of social workers much more to match needs, interests and preferences in family finding.
- Interference by birth family may prevent the child developing attachments to the adoptive parents.
- The creation of a general climate of insecurity may present problems.

- Adoptive parents might not feel in control of the situation.
- Abusive or harmful relationships between the birth child and birth relatives may be maintained in contact to the detriment of the child's wellbeing.

Contact and disabled children

The role of contact in promoting the emotional wellbeing of disabled children is often overlooked. It should never be assumed that children's impairments prevent them from understanding loss of links and therefore that contact has no significance. Face-to-face contact can help disabled children to make sense of their world and feel greater acceptance of themselves. However, careful preparation and support for contact are often required as the two sets of adults may be at different stages in their acceptance and feelings regarding of the child's difficulties (Argent 1996, 2003a).

Case example – contact for a disabled child

Joanne was adopted by a family who already had six disabled adopted and birth children. She could not walk, talk or hear. This was an open family with truly open adoptions. All birth relatives were welcome and came and went with varying regularity. Joanne's mother had moved to another country and letters were exchanged at Christmas and just before Joanne's birthday in July. Her father, a local teacher, visited every week and looked after Joanne for the evening to give the family a break. Then he started coming more often in the holidays and at some weekends. He liked being useful and the family was grateful for the help. One might have said that Joanne did not react to her father's visits but the adopters felt sure that she was calmer when he came and that she benefited from the good atmosphere when he was there. They said, 'On some level she knows. It doesn't have to be on our level, she finds her own level in her own world'.

Planning contact

The majority of contact arrangements for adopted children with members of their birth family involve indirect contact. Only a small proportion of adopted children are in face-to-face contact with their birth relatives (Rushton 2003a). When there is face-to-face contact, it is more often with birth brothers and sisters than with birth parents.

For any form of contact, effective planning and reviewing of contact arrangements, and the commitment of both the adoptive parents and birth relatives to making it work, contribute to making the contact a positive experience that meets the adopted child's needs. It is important that adoptive parents are supported in holding onto their parental authority and responsibility for deciding what is best for the child.

For contact to be emotionally safe, meaningful and purposeful for the adopted child, it has to be supported by an effective three-way relationship between the birth parents, adopters or special guardians, and the child or young person. In these circumstances, research suggests that if an adopted child has some contact with their birth family and it works well, it is better than where there is no contact at all. The absence of contact can present difficulties for all three parties – the child, the adoptive family and the birth relatives (Neil 2003).

It is important that realistic plans for contact are made at the Care Plan stage as over-optimistic arrangements can seriously affect family finding or set expectations about contact which adoptive parents find difficult to manage, whether it is indirect or face-to-face contact.

The birth parents ideally need to have reached an understanding of their future role with their adopted child as a 'non-parental parent' and be prepared to accept the alternative carers as the day-to-day parents, with all the implications. If they have managed this, then they will be unlikely to undermine the placement and contact may be in the interests of all parties. This may not happen immediately and it is important to keep the door open by ensuring, where possible, that adopters or special guardians get to meet birth parents at the outset and, where appropriate, are encouraged to remain in contact with them. This requires the support of professionals and is unlikely to happen otherwise.

If, on the other hand, they have not come to terms with the loss of their adopted child, then their influence on the child, who may already be torn by loyalty and worry over their wellbeing, may serve to prevent the child from benefiting from the placement and accepting the new carers. Contact is then likely to be contraindicated.

Contact once a child is placed

Contact can help an adopted child to settle into a new family. For example, for a child who has had to take responsibility for their birth parents, well-managed contact supported by adoptive parents which assures a child that a birth parent is well, can help them settle into an adoptive family (Neil 2002).

For some children, the loss, anxiety and guilt caused by having to relinquish important relationships may undermine the process of settling in a new family (Borland et al. 1991). Whether contact impacts negatively on the child's relationship with adoptive parents is likely to depend on the quality of such contact. If birth relatives express support for the adopted child in their new family, this can be important in helping children feel able to make new relationships. Some small-scale studies suggests that face-to-face contact does not have negative effects on adoptive parents feelings of parental authority, entitlement to parent or their sense of closeness to their adopted child (Neil 2002). Few studies have looked at later-placed children and the effects of contact over time on the stability of adoptive families.

In the context of a previously abusive relationship, an adopted child's refusal to have contact must always be taken seriously, because even indirect contact may recreate the abusive experience in the mind of the child. A balance has to be made between the child's wish for contact and the risk that contact may also undermine the placement.

Contact arrangements will need to be renegotiated over time owing to the changing developmental needs of the adopted child or changes in the adoptive or birth family circumstances and a family mediation model may be helpful in achieving this.

Indirect contact with a child's immediate birth family

Indirect contact is currently being built into more plans for adopted children and can work well in meeting the needs of the child for information about their birth family and is helpful for birth relatives who want to know about their child's wellbeing and development but mediated letter contact has been found to have disadvantages compared to more face-to-face contact, leading to more misunderstanding and people misinterpreting each other (Grotevant and McRoy 1998; Sykes 2000).

Birth parents may not understand their importance for their child, for example, as a source of information to help them find out who they are, as they are the only people who can answer certain questions. Children can feel that their birth parents do not care if they do not write.

Face-to-face contact with a child's immediate birth family

Difficulties between adopters and birth parents often concern issues of fear (related to birth family and fears of recrimination), anger and blame (that birth parents had neglected and caused damage to the adopted child), competition with birth parents, and empathy (especially for birth mothers). If adoptive parents have control and influence in contact arrangements their confidence as parents and commitment to contact can develop. Many adoptive and birth parents manage contact well without agency support (Sykes 2000).

Contact for older adopted children who have a relationship with their birth relatives may have the purpose of maintaining access to significant attachment figures in their past lives, while making sure they continue to feel secure about their place in their adoptive family. For them it may be important to have time with their birth relatives without their adoptive parent being present. This requires careful planning and support and a collaborative approach between the adoptive and birth families.

Birth parents can easily feel marginalised and judged negatively as a result of the process that led to their adopted child being adopted or cared for by special guardians. They may need helping in coping with loss, maintaining self-respect and staying connected with their adopted children. Sometimes birth relatives find it easier to be supported by staff in voluntary agencies who have special skills in working with birth parents and are not associated with the original process of the child's adoption (Charlton et al. 1998).

The adopters or special guardians may not have been prepared for contact with birth parents. They may find deterioration in the child following contact and this must be taken seriously. They need to be able to support the contact and if they are unable to do so, insistence on it may threaten the placement. If these negative attitudes persist, either the adoptive parents are right in their assessment of the negative impact on their adopted child, or they may not recognise their child's needs accurately.

Past difficulties may continue to be evident in contact meetings and the child can be left with a mixture of feelings leading to difficult behaviours. In this case, contact may be unhelpful to the adopted child's developing sense of their identity, especially if poorly managed and supported. This is especially problematic if birth parents remain unable to accept parenting role of the adopters or special guardians (Howe and Steele 2004).

Contact with birth brothers and sisters

Face-to-face contact with birth brothers and sisters forms part of many face-to-face contact arrangements, and research suggests that the majority of such arrangements work well and can be more straightforward than contact with birth parents (Macaskill 2002; Rushton et al. 2001). However, contact with birth brothers and sisters can be complex and requires careful assessment. The contact needs of one adopted child may well not be the same as their brothers and sisters and is often hard to know how to prioritise their different needs.

Case example – differing needs of brothers and sisters

Jo, a 9-year-old boy who had been the main carer for his younger brothers and sisters, very much wanted to have face-to-face contact with his 7-year-old adopted brother. Jo's memories of his brother were very strong and he was desperate to check and see how his younger brother was. Jo's adoptive parents felt this would be in his best interests. His younger brother had few memories of his older brother and no particular wish for contact. He was struggling with other issues in his placement and his adoptive parents felt that contact at this point was likely to unsettle him.

Complicated contact arrangements for adopted children from different birth families who are living together can be time-consuming and disruptive in a way that is not always thought through when contact plans are made.

Contact with members of the child's wider birth family

Wider family members may have provided protection and security in a context that has been highly unstable or disruptive. Birth grandparents, for example, may be important figures for children and young people and grandparental contact may be in the best interests of the child. Breaking off contact with wider family members who have provided some security may create a level of loss and disruption for children being placed for adoption and make it more difficult for them to become attached in their adopted family. The role of significant wider birth family members to an adopted child should be borne in mind when drawing up and reviewing contact arrangements and support for children and their families.

Other significant people in children's past lives

Adopted children have made significant connections with other adults in their past lives, such as previous foster carers, and can benefit from the continuity and affirmation which their contact can bring. The importance of recognising the potential significance of such people for a child's sense of identity and self-worth and continuity is reflected in the Welfare Checklist of the Adoption and Children Act 2002.

Developing 'adoption aware' services

Children who are adopted or cared for by special guardians have contact with a wide range of services including health, education and social services. It is essential that professionals working in those services are 'adoption aware', which means having an understanding of some of the specific issues facing children who are adopted or cared for by special guardians and their families, and how that affects the support and services they need. Staff in these services may require support and advice about adoption and special guardianship, so that they can provide the approach that is needed by the children and their families. In turn, adoptive families and special guardians may need support in establishing working relationships with staff from these and other services.

Assessment, training and support

The process of assessment, training for adoptive parenting and providing support to meet a specific child's needs should be viewed as an ongoing process rather than a series of events. It is easy to see the process as linear rather than developmental, following the stages of becoming an adoptive family. The assessment of adopters is a challenging task both for prospective adopters and adoption workers. Workers are required to carry out an in-depth Home Study, looking in part at the parenting capacities of the prospective adopters, and to convey, in preparation groups and associated events, something of the potential complexities of the task of adoptive parenting. This has often to be done with prospective adopters who do not have children of their own and who may find the realities of the hypothetical additional needs of adopted children hard fully to take on board. For prospective adopters, the process of assessment and the consideration of their application by the Adoption Panel and the agency decision maker is also often an emotionally charged time where the decision whether or not they are considered 'suitable to adopt' is uppermost in their minds.

Some agencies have shifted the emphasis of their assessment to a more 'child-led' approach whereby a potential link is made between prospective adopters and a child before some of the work of assessment, training and planning support is undertaken (Cousins 2003; Cousins 2006). This maybe through prospective adopters identifying children they would like to put themselves forward as carers for in the relevant adoption organisations publications. A number of agencies run schemes where prospective adopters are invited early on in the assessment process to a meeting where they are introduced to a range of children who need adoptive parents, through individual profiles, videos and posters made by the children and their foster carers and social workers (Lowe et al. 1999). Prospective adopters can express an interest in a specific child or children and may later be assessed for a link with those children. The process helps to engage and empower prospective adopters and allows the assessment process and the identification of required training and other support to be much more clearly focused on building up the capacity of the prospective adopters to meet the needs of a specific child.

Whatever the process, agencies and workers need to take into consideration when the offer of a specific piece of training or a package of adoption support might be best timed for a child and family.

Assessing adopted children's developmental needs using the *Assessment Framework*

Chapters 5, 6 and 7 identify the special areas for consideration when assessing the needs of adopted children and families, in each of the dimensions of the three domains:

- adopted children's developmental needs
- adoptive parenting capacity
- family and environmental factors.

This chapter focuses on adopted children's developmental needs. Chapter 6 looks at adoptive parenting capacity and Chapter 7 explores family and environmental factors that can affect adopted children's developmental needs and adoptive parenting capacity. In each chapter, the identification and assessment of needs or difficulties in each domain is often accompanied by an analysis of how they may relate to relevant dimensions in other domains. This is in order to illustrate common patterns of influence across the different domains of the child's developmental needs, parenting capacity and family and environmental factors in adoption and their relationship to possible plans for intervention or support. It should be borne in mind that, in practice, it is important to assess the three domains separately before analysing the connections, rather than jumping to conclusions about the patterns that may apply.

Case examples are used to illustrate particular points. Pointers for practice are provided for each dimension to assist workers in making assessments.

> *Assessment of what is happening to a child require that each aspect of a child's developmental progress is examined, in the context of the child's age and stage of development. Account must be taken of any particular vulnerability, such as a learning disability or a physically impairing condition, and the impact they may have on progress in any of the developmental dimensions. Consideration should also be given to the social and environmentally disabling factors hitch have an impact on the child's development, such as limited access for those who are disabled and other forms of discrimination. Children who have been maltreated may suffer impairments to their development as a result of injuries sustained and/or the impact of the trauma caused by their abuse. There must able a clear understanding of what a particular child is capable of achieving successfully at each stage of development, in order to ensure that he or she has the opportunity to achieve his or her full potential.*
>
> (DoH et al. 2000b: 18)

A holistic view of adopted children, which recognises both their needs and their strengths, is essential in providing a balanced picture of the child. All assessments of support needs, whether prior to placement or post-placement, should consider the child's history and experiences during the key phases of development (i.e. infancy, preschool, middle childhood and adolescence) to establish specific vulnerabilities they may have as a result of adverse experience and areas of resilience and strength which result from protective factors both in their birth family and subsequent placements in foster care or elsewhere.

Such an assessment helps to assess the likely support a child will need when placed for adoption. The balance of resilience and vulnerability will be different for each adopted child. Some children will have considerable needs and relatively little resilience. Others will have specific areas of need balanced by resilience in other areas. The capacity of the adoptive parents to respond to the specific needs of the child and the support they may require to do so can then be assessed. When a group of brothers and sisters are placed together it is not uncommon to find they have very different patterns of vulnerability and resilience.

In assessing the support needs when difficulties arise once a child is placed, it is helpful to use an approach where the use of screening tools are followed by specific enquiries about difficult areas and areas of strength.

Health

Health includes growth and development as well as physical and mental well being. The impact of genetic factors as well as of any impairment should be considered. Involves receiving appropriate health care when ill, an adequate and nutritious diet, exercise, immunisations where appropriate and developmental checks, dental and optical care and, for older children, appropriate advice and information on issues that have an impact on health, including sex education and substance misuse.

(DoH et al. 2000b: 19)

Assessing needs

Assessments of the adopted child's health needs should be multidisciplinary and multi-agency in order to gain a full picture of the child's current and future health needs and the support they are likely to require (Kelly et al. 2003).

Prior to placement, a full holistic assessment of a child's health is required (DoH 2002a; Farina et al. 2004; Mather 2003), in line with the statutory guidance, *Promoting Health for Looked After Children* (DoH 1999a). The adoption medical is an important starting point to assessing an adopted child's health needs. It should

- provide an accurate and realistic review of the child's physical health and development in the context of their social and emotional functioning
- include a comprehensive family medical history and a consideration of preventative health measures such as vision, hearing and dental checks.

For adopted children with complex health needs, it may be necessary for a community consultant paediatrician or the agency medical adviser to undertake particular aspects of the assessment (Beckett et al. 2003).

Prospective adoptive parents and professionals should have access to full and accurate health information on both the child and the birth family in order to make informed decisions about their capacity to care for a particular child and the support they may require.

The normal health history of the child is often incomplete, especially for adopted disabled children (Argent 2003a). For example, inoculations, dental care and developmental milestones may not be fully recorded. Continuity of knowledge about a child's health history is then lost and new parents have to cope with avoidable gaps in information. Medical records will need to be updated before a child is placed, to ensure that they are as full and accurate as possible.

Awareness of the specific health problems that adopted black and minority ethnic children may encounter is essential, for example sickle-cell anaemia and thalassaemia. The potentially damaging effect of racism and isolation on children's mental health also should be recognised. In inter-country adoption, particular difficulties can arise due to the frequent and significant gaps in the child's medical history, lack of health information about the birth parents and lack of an up-to-date, accurate and detailed assessment of their current health status. It is very important that all children entering the United Kingdom for adoption from overseas have a comprehensive health assessment as soon as possible after their arrival, so that information gaps can be filled and appropriate assessment and treatment needs identified.

The complex interplay between genetic and environmental factors should be considered in relation to the adopted child's development. Genes, to a large extent, determine physical characteristics, intellect, behaviour and predisposition to illness and disease (Turnpenny 1995). Learning disabilities in birth relatives, for example, are an important indicator of possible learning disabilities in adopted children (Scott and Lindsey 2003).

Genetic issues can prove to be complicated due to absence of information about birth family medical history (Grant 1995). When birth relatives will agree to having a medical of their own, some of these difficulties may be overcome (Mather 2003). Adopted children, parents and health and other professionals are disadvantaged if they do not have as full information as possible available to them about the child's genetic heritage.

There is some evidence that physical health matters and anxiety and depression may be overlooked when adopted children also have severe behavioural problems (Hill and Thompson 2003), and workers should be alert to this.

The *Strengths and Difficulties Questionnaire* gives screening information about emotional and behavioural problems and needs in children and young people from 3 to 16 (DoH et al. 2000a; Goodman 1997). It identifies difficulties with prosocial (sociable) behaviour, hyperactivity, emotional problems, conduct (behavioural) problems and peer relationship problems. There are questionnaires for adult caregivers, which can also be used by teachers, and for young people between the ages of 11 and 16. This can be used by younger children where they understand the questions. The *Adolescent Wellbeing Scale* can be used with adopted children and young people between 7 and 16 and asks about different aspects of their life

(Birleson 1980; DoH et al. 2000a). It enables workers to gain more understanding and insight on how an adopted adolescent feels about their life and their needs.

The agency medical adviser has a vital role in coordinating the collection of information, assessing health needs and providing advice and counselling to prospective new adoptive parents. Medical advisers are now required to provide a summary on a child's health in their Child Placement Report and on the health of prospective adopters as part of the report for panel under the Adoption and Children Act 2002 (DfES 2005c). There are sometimes delays in medical information being available to relevant health professionals when a child is placed for adoption or with special guardians. The adoption agency should ensure that medical records are transferred to the new GP as soon as possible after placement.

Care should be taken to involve adopted children and young people appropriately in discussions regarding their health needs (DoH 2002a) and their wishes should be taken into account.

Pointers for practice in health

- The pre-adoption health assessment is an important point at which to make a holistic assessment of the adopted child's current and future health needs.
- The medical records of looked after children should be as full and detailed as possible. Medical advisers can identify gaps and advise on possible ways of filling them.
- Workers and families should be aware that medical information may be incomplete. Families may benefit from or require support in managing uncertainties surrounding an adopted child's health.
- Medical information about an adopted child's birth relatives should as full as possible. Arranging for birth relatives to have a medical of their own may be helpful in this respect.
- It is important to identify any impairments an adopted child may have as early as possible so that plans can be made for their health and educational needs. Previous foster carers may be helpful sources of information.
- It is important to know as much detail as possible about any abuse, neglect, trauma, separations and loss a child has suffered, as this may affect their future health and development.
- Adopted children and young people should be involved in discussions and planning regarding their health needs.
- There should, at all times, be a holistic and coordinated response to health issues. The ASSA has a coordinating role in ensuring that services share relevant information.

Education

Education covers all areas of a child's cognitive development which begins from birth. Includes opportunities for play and interaction with other children, access to books, the development of skills and interests and the need to experience success and achievement. Involves an adult interested in educational activities, progress and achievements, who takes account of the child's starting point and any special educational needs.

(DoH et al. 2000b: 19)

Assessing needs

For adopted children placed at an early age, an assessment of cognitive development is important for assessing support needs. This will be based on information from sources such as the GP, health visitor and health centre etc. Knowledge of the Sheridan charts illustrating the developmental progress of infants and young children (DoH 2000a: 23) is useful in establishing the level of cognitive development of a child when placed and in tracking their progress during placement.

Prior to placement, workers should ensure that information from an adoptive child's previous school(s) is up to date, comprehensive and transferred in good time. The relevant statutory guidance, *The Education of Young People in Public Care* (DoH 1999b), sets out the government's expectations. Such information should include a personal education plan and, where relevant, a statement of special educational need, and details of speech therapy or other support received, which would form part of the child's Care Plan. Personal educational plans should be in place for all looked after children and form the basis for planning for educational needs after adoption (Fletcher-Campbell 2001).

If educational difficulties are apparent or predicted, an inter-agency approach is necessary. This often involves close work between adoption agency staff and educational staff in school. There should be careful exploration of the links between the child's history, the adoptive process and the child's educational needs. Adoptive parents may need help to decide what information about the child's background is appropriate for teachers, educational psychologists, school nurses and others to have to inform their assessments and develop effective strategies for support (DoH 2002b). Parents have to be sensitive to their child's wishes and feelings when judging what to disclose, even on a 'need to know' basis and decisions in this area are often finely balanced (Prior 2003).

Education is important for all children, including adopted children and especially those likely to experience discrimination. For black and minority ethnic children it is important to recognise that assessment tools used in school are often euro-centrically or American based. Black children, especially African Caribbean boys, are particularly vulnerable to bullying and also to teachers having low expectations of them, which can result in performance below their ability level and eventually their exclusion.

The *HOME Inventory* gives important information about the learning environment provided for the child and to observe how they are responding (Cox and Walker 2002; Joyce 2003). Items assessed include, for example, for 0–3 year olds the provision of play materials and opportunities for stimulation. Learning materials and language and academic stimulation for 3–6 year olds, and learning and leisure opportunities provided for 6–10 year olds. A *HOME Inventory* carried out in the birth family and then again in subsequent placements provides invaluable information about the support needs for children's cognitive development and education.

The *In My Shoes* (Calam et al. 2000) interview has a special module which allows the worker to explore with the child their experience of the whole school environment, including lessons, different aspects of the timetable, playtime, relationships with teachers and school friends and homework.

The *Family Assessment* (Bentovim and Bingley Miller 2001) allows the exploration of key factors that affect a child's cognitive development and education, including stimulation and encouragement, the nature of parent–child relationships and communication in the family.

For older adopted children, it is important to assess their adjustment to school and learning and the *Strengths and Difficulties Questionnaire* (DoH et al. 2000a; Goodman 1997) completed by the teacher, adoptive parents or child/young person gives a picture of the child in various contexts (home and school and with peers), their adjustment at school, their cognitive progress and whether there is a need for a specialist assessment, including statementing. They can also form the basis for opening up discussion with adoptive parents and children. The *Code of Practice for Special Educational Needs* (DfES 2002) sets out the circumstances, processes and inter-agency expectations in assessing special educational needs.

Case example – managing a child's emotional developmental delay

Assessment

Darren, a 5-year-old adopted boy with some developmental delay and health needs, was operating more like a 3 year old in terms of his ability to interact and play with his peers. He quickly got into trouble because, when other children approached him or wanted something from him he could hit out, and he soon became known as an aggressive or 'naughty' boy.

Support/intervention

Luckily because of his other special needs he had a special needs assistant (SNA) and was fully statemented – though not on the basis of his emotional needs. The SNA was sent on a training course to help her understand the needs of emotionally traumatised children and her task changed after the first term. Instead of focusing primarily on monitoring his health needs, she was able to be alongside the boy in a role similar to that of a parent helping their 2 year old integrate into a toddler group. He had missed a developmental stage which he therefore then needed to go through when he reached school.

Case example – managing the transition to secondary school

Assessment

Jane, an 11-year-old adopted girl in Year 7 in transition to secondary school had managed all right in a small primary school but her adoptive parents recognised that, at home, she operated in many ways like a much younger child. Within the first half term of secondary school she was unhappy, disorganised and unable to keep up with work, lost her primary school friends and contacts and refused to go to school. Because of early disruptions and changes in her life, managing the change to secondary school was extra difficult. She connected change with previous separation and abandonment and her insecure attachment style meant that she was unable to feel she could trust the new adults teaching her.

Support/intervention

She needed the support of a learning mentor within the school whom she could find at regular times when she felt lost and anxious. Regular meetings were set up between parents and school to allow the parents to understand the pattern of homework and the expectations and they reported on her reactions to school. Crucially, when homework became a battleground at home, specialist advice from CAMHS staff to the school and parents made it possible to negotiate a special programme of essential homework during the first year which reduced anxiety and conflict and allowed the child to learn to manage the complexities of life in a new school.

Pointers for practice in education

- An adopted child's cognitive development, subsequent progress and success or otherwise at school is a key element in the success of an adoptive placement.
- Adopted children's educational achievement is affected by their genetic inheritance and their past experiences of care. School difficulties may be linked to learning or other disabilities, or to earlier experiences of abuse or neglect or inconsistent parenting or to having many changes of school (and placement) prior to permanent placement. Full information about the adopted child's birth family and the care the child received helps to predict how he or she is likely to achieve at school and the help they may require.
- As with other children, it is important to ensure that adopted children's special educational needs are assessed appropriately and that any school they are due to attend can access their personal education plan prior to placement and where they have one, their statement of special educational needs.

- The ASSA and other workers have a role, where requested by adoptive parents, in liaising between adoptive parents and child, the school and the local education authority and for developing collaborative links between the different services involved.
- Having an education adviser in an adoption agency can be very helpful in providing consultation, liaison and support to all concerned regarding the provision of education for children being placed for adoption.

Emotional and behavioural development

Emotional and behavioural development concerns the appropriateness of response demonstrated in feelings and actions by a child, initially to parents and caregivers and, as the child grows older, to others beyond the family. Includes the nature and quality of early attachments, characteristic of temperament, adaptation to change, response to stress and degree of appropriate self-control.

(DoH et al. 2000b: 19)

Assessing needs

The assessment of an adopted child's emotional and behavioural needs should always occur within the context of what is considered 'normal' for a child of this age and stage of development.

When assessing needs prior to placement, information should be collected from previous assessments of the child to gain a picture of their emotional and behavioural development and particular areas of vulnerability and resilience. This needs to be understood in the context of their history including any maltreatment, trauma, separations and losses they have experienced.

Attachment, grief and loss are key issues for an adopted child prior to placement with an adoptive family. It is essential to assess a child's wishes and feelings about being adopted as part of preparing them for adoption and identifying the support they need to move on and settle into an adoptive family. Careful direct work with children is necessary for this taking time to get to know them. This assessment falls in two stages. First, the worker should ascertain how much the child understands about adoption in the context of their past history and what it might mean for them. Second, the child's wishes and feelings once they have been matched with a particular family should be determined. Children may develop a different level of understanding of the meaning of adoption for them and the reality of having a new adoptive identity, especially if they are older. At this stage children may go through a phase of emotional turmoil recognising and acknowledging their ambivalent feelings and reviewing their wishes about adoption. In *My Shoes* (Calam et al. 2000) provides an invaluable tool for helping children communicate about their experiences and their wishes and feelings about their experience of past families in which they have lived, including their birth family and foster families and of adoption and for assessing their understanding and current needs.

Workers aiming to help children communicate about their lives need to take considerable care to use approaches which take account of developmental and attachment processes and the impact which abuse, neglect, trauma and separations and losses can have on a child's capacity to understand and communicate about what has happened to them and what they think and feel about their experiences (Schofield 2005).

When assessing support needs in the context of difficulties arising post place-ment, it is helpful to start by exploring the concerns of adoptive parents. The 'mapping the problem' section of the *Family Assessment* (Bentovim and Bingley Miller 2001) can be useful because it systematically explores with the family the nature of the specific difficulties, how they arise and their impact on the adopted child and other family members. Enquiries are made about solutions that already have been tried and other current concerns of family members.

If it is already clear that an adopted child has serious attachment or other emotional or behavioural problems, taking a multi-agency approach at an early stage in the assessment of the child's and family's support needs is likely to be helpful. This will usually to involve social services, education and CAMHS. Part of the ASSA's role is to provide advice to parents or colleagues in their own or other agencies as to the referral of children with more serious difficulties to more specialist therapeutic services with specifically designed programmes to address these difficulties (Archer and Burnell 2003; Howe and Fearnley 2003).

It is important to get a clearer picture of the nature and level of the difficulties before deciding how best to proceed. Screening tools are helpful and the *Strengths and Difficulties Questionnaire* (DoH et al. 2000a; Goodman 1997) focuses directly on a child's prosocial behaviour (helpful behaviour towards others), hyperactivity, emotional problems, conduct (behavioural) and peer relationship problems. The *Adolescent Wellbeing Scale* (Birleson 1980; DoH et al. 2000a) highlights the impact of difficulties encountered by a young person on their friendships, classroom learning, home life and leisure activities.

Specific enquiry about key areas can help to establish the level of difficulty and whether a referral for specialist assessment and support is indicated. If there were a significant number of difficulties in one category or problems in several categories, this would indicate the need for a specialist referral. This can include asking whether the adopted child is affected by any of the following:

- *Physical*
  - is complaining of aches or pains, headaches and so on
  - has problems with sleep, for example getting to sleep, nightmares, waking up early
  - has problems with food, for example reluctant or excessive eating, exces-sively selective eating
  - is wetting, soiling, self-harming.

- *Cognitive*
  - is or is not able to function at school or nursery at a level normally expected for a child of their age and ability.

- *Emotional*
  - has worries, anxieties about separations or strikingly self-sufficient
  - has general anxiety, worries taking up a lot of time upsetting or interfering with their lives

- is getting depressed, has times being miserable, sad, unhappy, tearful, or grumpy and irritable, losing interest, not wanting to be alive
- has problems with overactivity or poor concentration
- has responses which seem to be associated with stressful and traumatic events, vivid memories, troubling dreams, upsets at being reminded, distant, alert or jumpy.

- *Behavioural*
  - displays awkward and troublesome behaviour, temper outbursts, deliberately annoying people, blaming others, refusal to acknowledge responsibility
  - displays behaviour which gets into trouble including any dangerous, aggressive or antisocial behaviour and sexual behaviour
  - has a behaviour pattern of arguing persistently or being defiant, wanting to take control, trying to take excessive responsibility for their brothers and sisters, is showing regressive or developmentally inappropriately adult behaviour, i.e. behaving in a way more appropriate to a younger or older child.

- *Social relationships*
  - has difficulties about being in social situations, new people or places
  - has difficulties with peer relationships and if they are isolated, for example unable to sustain a consistent and appropriate friendship, alone at playtimes
  - any reservations, difficulties about relating to people from their own racial background or in denying their difference.

Case example – identifying the support needs of a group of brothers and sisters

Assessment

Jonathan, Marie, Sarah and Robert, aged between 1 and 12, were brothers and sisters who were adopted together having been severely neglected physically and emotionally. Three years later, their schools raised concerns about the children being unhappy, aggressive and unkempt. A social work assessment found the adopters overwhelmed by the out-of-control behaviour of the children and their own financial problems. The adoptive mother was depressed. The children were confused and angry over why they had been adopted. Assessment revealed that when placed, the individual needs of the children had been underestimated due to the lack of attention to family history in terms of the trauma the children had suffered and the impact of the previously close relationship of the older children with their birth mother. There had also been a tendency for professionals to see the children's needs collectively rather than individually. Coupled with inexperienced adopters it was little surprise that they struggled to meet the children's considerable individual needs. Adoption support should have been built in from the start.

> ### Support/intervention
>
> Ongoing help from an experienced babysitter, therapeutic help for the older children targeted at the reason for their adoption, financial help and parenting advice work from a family centre led to gradual improvement.

Attachment difficulties

When assessing attachment difficulties it is crucial to draw on information as to the adopted child's early patterns of attachment (i.e. secure, insecure or disorganised) with birth relatives and subsequent carers.

There are different ways of defining what is meant by attachment disorder among researchers, members of the medical profession and other professionals working with this group of adopted children and young people. but all would agree that there are some core features of attachment-disordered behaviour. Most significantly, for a young child, this would require careful observation of how the child interacts with a stranger. Unfortunately no established observational protocols have been validated to formally assess attachment disordered behaviour (O'Connor and Zeanah 2003), but for the purposes of identifying whether there are some attachment difficulties, a combination of good observation, Fahlberg's (1994) *Observation Checklists*, the *HOME Inventory* (Cox and Walker 2002) and the *Family Assessment* (Bentovim and Bingley Miller 2001) can all be helpful. *In My Shoes* (Calam et al. 2000) can be used to gain an understanding of the pattern of the child's attachments in their birth or foster family and later with their adoptive family.

Once the adopted child has been placed, it is helpful first to find out from the adoptive parents their account of the way attachments have developed and with whom, including wider family members. In particular, we need to establish how the child responds to separations and reunions, the pattern of who they seek comfort from when distressed or frightened, how they relate to people they do not know, and how they are before, during and after any contact with birth relatives.

Fahlberg's (1994) *Observation Checklists* provide a useful guide to assessing both the attachment behaviours and the responses of caregivers for children from infancy to adolescence. The checklists ask questions about the attachment related behaviour that might be expected to occur in the first year of life, the pre school years, middle childhood and teens. They similarly explore the level of responsiveness and sensitivity being demonstrated by the caregiver. The degree of 'fit' between the two can then be assessed and possible ways of increasing attunement may be considered. For instance, a question about a child aged under 1 year is whether he/she shows an interest in the human face and for the caregiver, whether he/she engages in face-to-face contact with the child. If this is not occurring, games, songs, rhymes and toys that encourage this sort of interaction might be suggested.

For preschool children, the checklists acknowledge that attachment behaviours will be centred on the relationship with the primary caregivers. Ways in which the child can communicate feelings and the degree to which the caregiver is attuned and responsive to this communication form the focus of the checklists. In middle childhood, there is recognition that the child's world is expanding beyond the family boundary to include school, peers and other adults. However, the connection between the child's behaviours and the response of the caregiver remains central. For example the questions 'Does the child show pride in accomplishments? Try new tasks? Exhibit confidence in own abilities?' can be matched with observations about whether the caregiver shows interest in the child's accomplishments, assigns the child age-appropriate responsibilities and comments on positive behaviours as well as negative ones. If there is a shortfall in the caregiver's responses, this might be explored and suggestions for adjustment might be agreed

Administering the *HOME Inventory* gives an opportunity, during an hour's interview, to gain an idea of the attachment patterns between adopted child and the main caregiver, and how the child responds to their care. This is obtained both through observation and by the detailed exploration with the adoptive parent of a specific day in the life of the child.

The *Family Assessment* looks at the nature of attachments in the family, including the pattern of care-seeking behaviour of the adopted child and caregiving by the adoptive parent. The ways emotions are expressed and responded to and whether relationships are supportive and valuing is also explored. This helps to establish how far an adopted child has been able to develop new attachments and where areas of difficulty lie.

Case example – an adoptive parent caring for a boy with a severe sleep disturbance

Assessment

Nathan, a 6-year-old boy, had been sexually abused in his birth family and removed at the age of 4 years. His first foster carer had commented on his difficulty in settling at night but in his second placement, where he shared a room with a younger child, this had seemed to improve. One year after his placement for adoption his adoptive mother, Diane, a single parent, was completely exhausted because Nathan would not settle at night until 11pm or 12am. For three to four hours he would shout and scream if he was left alone in his room. The only way he would go to sleep was if Diane actually stayed in his room and lay on his bed beside him without moving. She had tried various behavioural techniques such as gradually moving from lying by him, to staying in a chair by him, to being by the bedroom door etc. but it seemed that Nathan's anxiety about being alone in his room was too great to allow this to work. Diane had an older birth son of her own aged 11 years who was distressed by Nathan's screams and complaining because he never saw his mum in the evening, she wasn't there to help him with homework any more. Diane was near to calling social services to ask them to take Nathan back into care.

Her GP prescribed a mild sedative for Nathan at bedtime, which reduced the screaming, but not his anxiety about being alone.

Support/intervention

Diane eventually rang the adoption-placing agency to ask for help. She thought they would think that she was failing with Nathan, but instead they began to think about how they could help her. They suggested paying an experienced foster carer four nights a week to help with the bedtime routine thus allowing Diane some evening time with her birth son. This has been very helpful for Diane but Nathan still becomes acutely anxious at bedtime. The post-adoption worker referred Nathan to the local CAMHS team who she liaised with. They agreed a trial of medication, which is helping him to experience what it feels like to be calm and safe when falling asleep. The combination of the immediate resource of practical help from social services and the medical help from the local CAMHS services is helping Diane feel less alone and well supported with Nathan's problem.

Pointers for practice in emotional and behavioural development

- Adopted children's experiences of abuse and neglect and poor parenting or exposure to domestic violence are likely to affect their emotional and behavioural development and assessments for adoption support needs to be linked with earlier assessments of the child and birth family.
- Preparation of adopters should include training about the impact of early attachment difficulties and experiences of abuse, neglect and poor parenting on adopted children over time.
- Workers should gather as detailed and accurate information as possible about the adopted child and their background and an understanding of both the strengths and risks associated with the child's past life experiences.
- Adoptive parents should always be given accurate and full information about an adopted child's background and history presented in a way which makes clear links to the potential implications for a child's emotional and cognitive development and the difficulties they may encounter.
- Adoptive parents need to be aware that this information will never be complete and everyday family life may trigger traumatic memories for an adopted child.
- An adopted child's attachment history is particularly important in understanding any current attachment difficulties. Children often repeat their early attachment behaviours when they begin to settle into an adoptive family.
- Adopted children often develop significant attachments to foster carers which need to be taken account of in planning support for transitions. On the other hand, some insecure attachment behaviours by children towards

their foster carers are sometimes mistaken as evidence of more secure attachments.

- Adoptive parents may require help in identifying and understanding an adopted child's attachment behaviours and patterns in the context of the child's previous significant attachment experiences, and in developing strategies for helping a child develop more secure attachments.
- In assessing current and past emotional and behavioural difficulties workers should be aware that even when there has been treatment in the past, the effects of previous traumatic and stressful events may re-present at later developmental stages and may require further therapeutic intervention, particularly in adolescence.
- There are a number of ways workers can support adoptive parents in building up adopted children's resilience.
- Adoption support may include practical support and guidance or more specialist help for adoptive parents and children.

Identity

Identity concerns the child's growing sense of self as a separate and valued person. Includes the child's view of self and abilities, self image and self esteem and having a positive sense of individuality. Race, religion, age, gender, sexuality and disability may all contribute to this. Feelings of belonging and acceptance by family, peer group and wider society, including other cultural groups.

(DoH et al. 2000b: 19)

Assessing needs

When undertaking an assessment, in preparation for placement of the support a child may require, it is important to have an idea of the adopted child's likely sense of identity based on what is known about their experience in their birth family and subsequently. For children with a minority ethnic background, for example, it is essential to assess how their heritage in terms of race and ethnicity, their preferred language and any specific spiritual needs can be supported in a new adoptive family and how links with their birth family can be best maintained (Charlton et al. 1998; Harris 2005).

A child's identity and view of themselves will differ if they have been the object of emotional rejection, physical abuse or neglect. An adopted child who has been sexually abused may see themselves as being responsible for evoking a sexual response and a child who has been frequently punished is likely to see themselves as 'bad'. Alternatively a child can feel special as a result of a 'traumatic bond', e.g. if they have been related to as a partner or parental figure by their own birth parent. Assessing these patterns helps to identify a child's likely identity needs, and the support they will require. In subsequent placements and later, in the adoptive family, it will be easier to track whether a child's sense of themselves has altered.

Where identity issues arise for the child post-adoption, we need to understand the balance between the adopted child being seen as a member of their adoptive family and respected as an individual in the light of their special needs. The *Family Assessment* (Bentovim and Bingley Miller 2001) can help to assess how an adopted child is developing as an individual, their self-assertiveness and autonomy, and the degree of emotional involvement and sense of 'togetherness' as an adoptive family. Looking at the expectations and quality of the relationships between the adoptive parents and the adopted and other children, and between the children, helps to build up a picture of how an adopted child's identity needs are being responded to and where support may be needed.

Adopted children's needs to find out about their identity

Adopted children's need to ask questions about identity and capacity to understand the answers will vary as they develop. Assessment should consider the child's expressed needs in relation to asking and answering these questions, and should also anticipate the child's future needs. The resources available in finding answers to identity questions should also be considered, especially the amount, type, accuracy and tone of information available to the child about their background and the circumstances necessitating their adoption.

Lifestory books, memorabilia and other personal items are a key part of helping an adopted child develop their sense of identity. It is often helpful to review the lifestory book and quality of the information available with the adoptive parents to see the child's response, whether any recent life events and new information about the child's birth family have been added. Adoptive parents may value support in helping to use a lifestory book as part of responding to a child's identity needs.

The *In My Shoes* (Calam et al. 2000) interview allows the worker to explore with the child a range of settings in which they have lived and pictures and narrative generated during the interview can be printed out for the child.

Older adopted children and young people also may want to search for birth parents with whom they are not in touch. This is an extremely emotionally significant action for all concerned and it is important to assess the possible impact of both the process and the potential outcomes on all concerned. Adopted young people under the age of 18 years may not have access to their adoption files without the consent of their adoptive parents. If a search proceeds, it is important to consider the support needs of each party to maximise the chances of the process being a positive one.

Case example – promoting a positive sense of identity through indirect contact

Assessment

Mary, a 14-year-old girl, was placed for adoption as a baby with very little information about her birth parents and no photographs. As she developed into adolescence she became aware that she was physically very different from her adoptive family and she became negatively preoccupied with her physical shape. It became obvious that one of her needs was to know more about her birth family, in particular to find physical resemblance and place her identity into her birth family context.

Support/intervention

The adoption agency agreed to contact the birth parents. When the girl received information and photograph from her birth mother, she was immediately able to see a physical resemblance. The experience significantly helped to raise her self-esteem.

Pointers for practice in identity

- Adoptive parents and adopted children, need clear and accurate information about the child's past, including access to any new information that becomes available. Information may need to be searched out at a later stage depending on the developing identity needs of children, e.g. as they get older or more curious.
- Parents may need support in deciding how to share a child's birth family background and adoption story, especially when there is painful information. This may need to be part of the adoption support component of the Placement Plan.
- Maintaining existing activities and hobbies which they have enjoyed, and developing new ones as their interests and talents become clear, help an adopted child to build a positive sense of their identity. Support for families with an adopted disabled child will include helping parents to advocate for access to places a child wants to go and the provision of appropriate services and support to enable them to participate.
- Adopted young people may wish to make contact with their birth parents at a later stage. There is a role for ASSAs to liaise between the parties when requested and to ensure everyone concerned has the support they need.
- Black and minority ethnic adopted children and young people face particular challenges in relation to developing a sense of their ethnic and cultural identity, as they have to integrate the experience of being a member of two potentially marginalised groups. This is also true for disabled children. Workers may need to help these children and their families to understand the impact of discrimination and/or racism, as well as adoption.
- Children and young people who have been adopted by a family with a different cultural or racial identity to their own can feel particularly isolated. Families may need support in developing parenting strategies, finding out more about the child's ethnic and cultural heritage and making contact with people in the relevant communities.

- Adopted young people can find it helpful to meet with other adopted black or minority ethnic young people in a similar situation.
- Older adopted young people may require help with searching and reunion with their birth family. This is an emotionally challenging process and all concerned may need support.

Family and social relationships

Family and social relationships concern the development of empathy and the capacity to place self in someone else's shoes. Includes a stable and affectionate relationship with parents or caregivers, good relationships with siblings, increasing importance of age appropriate friendships with peers and other significant persons in the child's life and response of family to these relationships

(DoH et al. 2000b: 19)

Assessing needs

Creating a series of genograms and ecomaps (DoH 2000a) to reflect the adopted child's important family and social relationships over time in the different contexts in which they have lived helps to assess whether there are relationships within the birth family, including significant attachments, which it would be of value for the child to maintain and the support that might be required to do so. Conversely, concerns about retraumatising a child if contact were maintained may emerge. This provides the basis for more effective planning for the child and adoptive family's shorter and longer-term support needs.

Successful family and social relationships are based on the bedrock of a network of secure attachments. Conversely, difficulties in family and social relationships are often related to a pattern of insecure attachments for the adopted child. When problems with family and social relationships arise in an adoptive placement there are a number of ways of assessing the current vulnerabilities and protective factors for the adopted child as a basis for planning support.

The *Strengths and Difficulties Questionnaire* helps to assess the adopted child's relationships with peers including their friendships and leisure activities and to see how they are perceived at home and at school (DoH et al. 2000a). The *Family Activity Scales* look at joint child-centred family activity and support for independent activities (DoH et al. 2000a). The *Adolescent Wellbeing Scale* helps identify adopted young person's own perceptions of family and social relationships (DoH et al. 2000a). The family alliances section of the *Family Assessment* looks at strengths and difficulties in various family relationships, e.g. whether the adoptive parents are supportive, engaged and responsive towards the children or whether there is a degree of rejection, disqualification or avoidance (Bentovim and Bingley Miller 2001). The degree of affiliation and affection as against rivalry, competition, fighting or isolation between brothers and sisters can bee explored. The *HOME Inventory* also gathers information about parent–child interaction and involvement and the child's contact with other family members and the extended family (Cox and Walker 2002). *In My Shoes* enables a child to communicate about their experience of family and social relationships and how they feel about those close or not so close to them (Calam et al. 2000).

Where there are concerns about an adopted child facing discrimination and marginalisation as a result of their adopted status, the impact of this on their family and social relationships should be considered. They may also be facing attitudes which are racist, homophobic or sexist or which discriminate against disabled people. It is important to find out whether a child is able to mix with a range of peers including children who face the same challenges (Richards and Ince 2000), for example adopted disabled children, or children from back and minority ethnic groups, as this may help to identify specific support needs.

Case example – managing a child's response to trauma

Assessment

Harry, a 6-year-old adopted boy, was generally managing school quite well, but from the time he started school aged 5, he had regular occurrences of seriously losing control – sitting under a table in hunched-up position, screaming and running out of the classroom and sometimes out of the school. This behaviour was a result of traumatic abuse Harry had experienced as a much younger child. Staff were disturbed by the behaviour and sought advice. It was agreed that the behaviour reflected times when Harry was being overwhelmed with feelings he couldn't verbalise and that he needed containment and removal from the classroom.

Support/intervention

With the agreement of the adoptive parents, the staff devised a plan whereby, when Harry had an outburst, he was removed from the classroom and taken to a quiet room and held safely by a known member of staff until he was settled enough to return to the classroom. Over a period of time the outbursts reduced as Harry felt that the adults would keep him safe. This strategy required all members of staff to understand how the experiences of early trauma sometimes leads to apparently inexplicable bouts of behaviour over which the child has no control. Staff needed training to understand and accept the needs of the child and the head teacher needed to give permission for the time and resources required to handle the situation.

Pointers for practice in family and social relationships

- A child's Care Plan should include accurate information about, and assessment of, the pattern of family and social relationships, including significant attachments and those which provided a child with support and protection, so that adoptive parents and workers can develop informed strategies to help a child with relationship difficulties.
- Adopted children may have lived in birth or other families where the pattern of relationships was distressing or where their needs were not met. Parents may need support to understand and manage adopted children's behaviour when it reflects and repeats their attempts to adjust to earlier family relationships and insecure attachments.
- Workers should recognise that some troubled adopted children will find it difficult to join in the usual range of age-appropriate social activities.
- Developing positive family and social relationships is central to an adopted child's sense of self-worth and their capacity to develop social relationships in later life. Adoptive families may need support and advice in helping a child to develop a network of secure attachments and to build up school and local social relationships and develop their range of activities and interests.

Social presentation

Social presentation concerns the child's growing understanding of the way in which appearance, behaviour and any impairment are perceived by the outside world and the impression being created. Includes appropriateness of dress for age, gender, culture and religion; cleanliness and hygiene; and availability from parents or caregivers about presentation in different settings.

(DoH et al. 2000b: 19)

Assessing needs

Adopted children have often lived with several families in the past, including their birth family, and have had multiple influences and expectations in terms of appearance, culture, religion and other aspects of social presentation. Children's growing sense of how to present themselves socially is affected by their past experience which has to be understood it order to assess their support needs effectively.

Adopted children who have been rejected or neglected will have a poor sense of themselves, especially if there have been issues around poor cleanliness and hygiene and inappropriate dress which are likely to be associated with negative social presentation. Clearly it is an area of vulnerability for children if they have adapted to a particular negative presentation of themselves due to the standard of care they have received.

Tracking the progress of the child into the adoptive placement helps to assess whether the adopted child has a growing acceptance of more positive ways of presenting themselves, or whether they are continuing to have difficulties in this area and to assist adoptive families in working out strategies for helping the child.

Discussion of the answers given by adopted children and adults to the prosocial scale of the *Strengths and Difficulties Questionnaire* (DoH et al. 2000a) will provide information about the child's behaviour towards others and their understanding of its impact.

Assessing and tracking the particular needs of adopted children from black and minority ethnic groups, regarding, for example, their dress, appearance, care of their hair and specific cultural or religious identity needs. This can be especially important when they are placed with adoptive families from a different cultural or ethnic background. Appropriate support can be then be planned for the adoptive child and family where required.

When difficulties arise, consider the ways in which the adoptive parents have been able to promote their adopted child's satisfactory social presentation in the light of their specific needs and earlier vulnerabilities, and where they are encountering difficulties. This includes whether children have been able to adjust sufficiently to aspects of social presentation to help them feel comfortable in presenting themselves as a member of their new family, e.g. dress, ways of relating to others, style of talking.

The assessment may involve establishing the nature of any difficulties the child has over 'telling' others about their adopted status. Adopted children and their adoptive parents may need support with process of helping the child develop a way of talking about being adopted to others, when they wish to and in a manner which feels comfortable to them. This is especially important where an adopted child has visible differences from their adoptive family, e.g. when a black child is placed with a family from a different ethnic background, because this increases the pressure for the child and family.

The adoptive family life cycle chart (see Chapter 4) can be used to look at how successfully the adoptive family and adopted child are negotiating the various tasks related to helping a child with their social presentation. The *Family Assessment* helps identify how the family are adapting to the changing needs of the child as he or she settles in and becomes a member of the family (Bentovim and Bingley Miller 2001). The *HOME Inventory*, especially for 6–10 year olds, examines the opportunities for social contact and leisure opportunities available for the child, how the child is being encouraged to develop social responsible and mature behaviour and how the child is responding to the family (Cox and Walker 2002; Joyce 2003).

Pointers for practice in social presentation

- The transition for an adopted child of adapting their social presentation to a new family context can be a slow process depending on the child's earlier history and needs. The adoptive family life cycle chart can help to assess progress and to identify difficulties (see Table 4.1, p. 38).
- Adopted children may have concerns about how to present their adopted status to their peers and others and have difficulties in knowing how to talk about being adopted.

- The issues for children about adoption and how they present this aspect of themselves socially will change as they grow older.
- Children who are 'different' in other ways as well as being adopted, e.g. they have learning or physical impairments, may face extra difficulties in learning about how to present themselves socially.
- Parents may require support and advice about how to help adopted children to develop a narrative or 'story' about being adopted and deal with the reactions they may encounter.
- Children may need specialist help if they have serious concerns or problems with acknowledging or managing their adopted status.
- An important part of support services can be to enable adopted children and their adoptive families to meet socially and informally.

Self-care skills

Self-care skills concerns the acquisition by a child of practical, emotional and communication competencies required for increasing independence. Includes early practical skills of dressing and feeding, opportunities to gain confidence and practical skills to undertake activities away from the family and independent living skills as older children. Includes encouragement to acquire problem-solving approaches. Special attention should be given to the impact of a child's impairment and other vulnerabilities, and on social circumstances affecting the development of self-care skills.

(DoH et al. 2000b: 19)

Assessing needs

There are ranges of aspects of an adopted child's self-care that may require addressing in terms of adoption support. Knowledge of the pattern of normal child development is an important context for assessing an adopted child's self-care needs (see DoH 2000a).

Assessing an adopted child's vulnerabilities and areas of resilience in developing self-care skills, based on an understanding of their early history and their response to subsequent care, helps to identify the support they require. A child who has been seriously neglected, for example, may have a low level of self-care skills and need help to develop self-care skills.

Having to take a significant level of responsibility for younger brothers and sisters can affect a child's developing self-care skills and the impact of this should be assessed carefully. It is important to look at the cultural context as part of this assessment. In many black communities, caring for brothers and sisters is viewed as good practice and there is some evidence it can help children develop resilience. But some children, however, have had to be more self-sufficient than suited their needs and they may require support in relinquishing their expectation of having to look after others.

If there are still difficulties once an adopted child is with their adoptive family, they or their adoptive parents may require further support. In talking an adoptive parent and child through a specific day, using the *HOME Inventory* (Cox and Walker 2002), a range of self-care skills such as washing, dressing, mealtimes, getting to school are systematically explored. This helps to assess the areas of difficulty, the adoptive parents' adaptation to the child's specific needs and the extent to which the child is encouraged to develop appropriate self-care skills.

Pointers for practice in self-care skills

- Self-care can be an area where adopted children need special help. This may be because they have lived in family contexts where they did not learn self-care skills appropriate to their age and stage of development, or because they have had to take inappropriate levels of responsibility for caring for others – for their brothers and sisters or birth parents for example.
- Parents may require support and guidance in helping an adopted child develop self-care skills and confidence that matches their age and stage of development. This might focus on planning the steps towards greater independence for a particularly dependent child, or, alternatively, helping a child let go of their sense of responsibility for their brothers and sisters, for example.
- Occasionally adoptive parents unrealistic expectations of adopted children may mean they inadvertently support an unhelpful pattern of self-care in a child, for example, by encouraging them to remain dependent, or supporting an over-responsible child in caring for younger children. Parents may need help in looking at the impact on the child's development and developing alternative approaches.
- Adopted disabled children and their families may require specialist services, financial assistance and equipment to promote the child's self-care skills and ASSAs have a liaison and coordinating role in ensuring they have access to the services and resources they need.
- Because of their early experience, learning life skills may be a challenging developmental task for older adopted children, and adoptive parents and young people may benefit from advice and access to groups and other resources to help young people learn to be independent.

Chapter 6

Assessing adoptive parenting capacity using the *Assessment Framework*

This chapter looks at adoptive parenting capacity and some of the special parenting skills that can be required to provide for the needs of adopted children.

> *Critically important to a child's health and development is the ability of parents and caregivers to ensure that the child's developmental needs are being appropriately and adequately responded to, and to adapt to his or her changing needs over time.*

(DoH et al. 2000b: 20)

There are many rewards in adoptive parenting and an important focus of adoption support is to help adoptive parents and appreciate the positive in a child, and child's achievements even if at times they are small. Adoptive parents and special guardians offer parenting to children who have not been born into their family, many of whom have experienced early adversity and all have suffered some damage to their attachments. The additional parenting tasks and challenges involved require enhanced parenting skills or 'parenting plus', resilience and considerable emotional resources. In a small but significant number of cases, the additional needs of an adopted child will be extreme and adoptive parents may find their skills and energies stretched to the limit.

It is likely that all adoptive parents and special guardians will need some level of support at one or more stages of their adoptive family life cycle and, in some cases, the requirements will be varied and ongoing. The accurate assessment of support needs is a key task. The primary aim of assessment is to identify, alongside adoptive parents, the areas where they may need help and then to identify the type of support or services that will best meet their needs. It is important that adoptive parents understand, from the outset, the likelihood that their adopted child will have some additional needs and that the provision of support is not a reflection on their parenting.

Three factors have been associated with predicting breakdown in foster care that are likely to be relevant to the adoption context (Sinclair 2002). These are parental lack of confidence, behavioural problems in the child and a lack of 'click' by which adoptive parents feel they do not understand or are not getting on with the child. These factors should be carefully considered at the point of matching and when assessing support needs.

When adoptive families request assessment post-placement

It is important for parenting difficulties to be identified at the earliest possible stage when they arise in a placement. This argues for continuity of support worker who will know the family well and be able to work from a position of trust. Consumer studies make it clear that all adoptive families value a dependable, consistent relationship with a support worker who they feel knows them well, is knowledgeable on the issues that pertain to them and their adopted child and who cares about them and their child (Sellick et al. 2004).

When adoptive parents request support later in placement, it is important to be sensitive to their needs and difficulties. Parenting a traumatised child can have a serious impact on parental and family relationships and the self-confidence and self-esteem of adoptive parents can be severely undermined (Burnell 2003). Parents may need help and encouragement to look after their own needs as well as those of their child. An awareness of the nature of the long-term impact of early trauma in completing such assessments is essential (Archer and Gordon 2004; Beek and Schofield 2004b).

Therefore a key focus of this book is identifying the support needs of adoptive parents and special guardians and meeting them so that they can continue to respond to the developmental needs of their children. In some cases, this might mean helping adoptive parents to enhance their parenting capacity or to learn new skills or approaches to parenting. However, in a very small number of cases, assessments of the support services require may provide evidence that adoptive parents do not have the capacity to provide for their adopted child's needs, whatever the quantity or quality of support offered, and in such cases the likelihood of the child suffering significant harm may need to be assessed.

The use of the Assessment Framework assessment tools in assessing parenting capacity

There is a range of assessment tools that specifically focus on parenting and help to identify strengths and areas of difficulty in parenting and the support adoptive parents need to provide the enhanced parenting adopted children often require. The *Parenting Daily Hassles Scale* (DoH et al. 2000a) helps to assess the frequency, intensity and impact on the parents of a range of daily parenting experiences which can be a 'hassle' to parents, e.g. mealtimes, babysitters, behaviour in public, quarrels with brothers or sisters. The behaviours rated are often particularly challenging with adopted children and it provides a user-friendly and valuable way identifying parenting problems which may require adoption support. The *HOME Inventory* (Cox and Walker 2002) covers all key areas of the parenting capacity domain and the *Family Assessment* (Bentovim and Bingley Miller 2001) looks at promoting development: stimulation, emotional warmth and praise, the nature of attachments and guidance care and management of the children.

Basic care

Basic care involves providing for the child's physical needs, and appropriate medical and dental care. Includes the provision of food, drink, warmth and shelter, clean and appropriate clothing and adequate personal hygiene.

(DoH et al. 2000b: 21)

Understanding the adopted child's previous history of caregiving and the possible links with the current difficulties may help make sense of the child's behaviour and give an indicator of whether the child and family need specialist advice and guidance about how provide for the basic care needs of the child.

For adoptive parents of adopted children who are disabled, the amount of time and the physical and emotional energy required for basic care will need to be assessed, along with the range of resources available to the parents.

Using the *HOME Inventory* to talk through a specific but typical day gives the opportunity to assess whether the child's basic care needs are being met and any specific difficulties adoptive parents may be having in adapting to the child's extra needs. These often relate to a rage of factors, including earlier adverse experiences, e.g. a severely neglected child wanting to eat and eat and not knowing when to stop, the considerable basic care needs a child with physical impairments may have, or the struggles over everyday basic care tasks such as feeding, washing, dressing which adoptive parents may have with children with insecure attachments. Adoptive parents may need support to develop strategies for responding to these difficulties, and may need referral for specialist help if the difficulties are severe.

Pointers for practice in basic care

- If there are difficulties over basic care, it is useful to assess how far the adopted child's specific basic care needs are being met, the nature of any difficulties and how the adoptive parents understand them, what the barriers are to the adoptive parents being able to modify their responses and the support they need to be able to do so.
- Adoptive parents may need guidance about how to meet their adopted child's specific basic care needs. Financial support, practical help or short breaks may also be appropriate.
- Adopted children who have had experience of neglect or very poor parenting may well not have had their basic care needs met and this can affect their development, and their response to the provision of adequate care in an adoptive family, which can present challenges for their adoptive parents.
- Adoptive parents may benefit from exploration of shared understandings of the adopted child's history caregiving and known or possible maltreatment and considering the possible links with current difficulties.
- Even to provide basic care for some adopted children can be a major problem and specialist support may needed. This is especially the case with children with attachment difficulties, where adoptive parents find struggles over everyday care, e.g. dressing, food, washing, can become a major battleground because of the child's need to try to take control of every aspect of their day-to-day life.

Ensuring safety

Ensuring safety involves ensuring a child is adequately protected from harm or danger. It includes protection from significant harm or danger, and contact with unsafe adults/other children and from self-harm. Recognition of hazards and danger both in the home and elsewhere.

(DoH et al. 2000b: 21)

Ensuring the safety of an adopted child is sometimes a particularly challenging task and the potential support that adoptive parents may require can be assessed on the basis of a full understanding of the child's early experiences of abuse and neglect for example, or their attachment difficulties. An assessment of the adoptive parent's understanding of the reasons for the extra care needed to keep their child safe and the actions needed to promote their safety and protection may reveal they need advice and training prior to placement, or if difficulties arise at a later stage.

Once an adopted child is in placement, there are a range of behaviours which adoptive parents may have difficulties with that can put a child in potential unsafe situations. This could for example include over-trusting (with strangers) or sexualised behaviour by a child, running away, drug or alcohol misuse. It is important to assess both the level and nature of the child's needs regarding their safety, the capacity of the parent to understand and respond to those needs and the nature of the support that they may require to do so. The parenting component of the *Family Assessment* (Bentovim and Bingley Miller 2001) can help to highlight strengths and difficulties in the nature of attachments in the family and the protection, care and management of children.

Pointers for practice in ensuring safety

- Ensuring a child's safety is a universal task for parents but one that often has particular relevance for children who have been permanently separated from their birth families.
- Adopted children who have received poor parenting or been actively abused often have difficulties in recognising dangerous situations and seeking the care they need.
- Considerable parenting skills are required to make sure some adopted children are safe, and adoptive parents need detailed information about a child's previous adverse experiences, and the pattern of caregiving they have received, to be able to respond appropriately to the child's needs. They may need support and help to develop strategies to keep their child safe.
- Adopted children, who have been sexually abused and/or seriously neglected will have developed patterns of behaviour which potentially place them at risk, sometimes including the way they relate to adoptive family members. Parents may not have the necessary skills to manage the child's behaviour and need specialist help to do so.
- Adopted children with insecure avoidant attachment patterns, are likely to have learnt not to seek the care and help they need from their attachment figures when they are in danger or distressed. If difficulties are persistent

in adoptive parents knowing how best to respond to a child's needs, especially if they relate to a child's attachment history or experiences of abuse and neglect, then specialist help may be required.

- Special care should be taken with some adopted children with learning disabilities to ensure they are kept safe because they do not always recognise physical or other dangers, and disabled children are more at risk of being abused. Parents may need and value advice on how to approach issues of safety, while also encouraging independence.

Emotional warmth

Emotional warmth includes ensuring that the child's emotional needs are met and giving the child a feeling of being especially valued and a positive sense of his or her own racial and cultural identity. Includes ensuring the child's requirements for secure, stable and affectionate relationships with significant adults, with appropriate sensitivity and responsiveness to the child's needs. Appropriate physical contact, comfort and cuddling sufficient to demonstrate warm regard, praise and encouragement.

(DoH et al. 2000b: 21)

Adopted children with attachment difficulties and who have experienced separations and losses can be challenging to parent and adoptive parents may find it hard to provide the emotional responsiveness their adopted child needs. In assessing the support of adoptive parents may require it is useful to map how a child has responded to previous differing experiences of emotional responsiveness, for example, in their birth family compared to skilled and attuned foster carers, to predict the particular quality of emotional relatedness the child is likely to need and how to support adoptive parents in providing that.

Caring for an adopted child who is unresponsive or rejecting emotionally can prove extremely exhausting, frustrating and depressing for adoptive parents and part of the assessment involves identifying the level of difficulty the adoptive parents are experiencing to see whether they might benefit from specialist support. It can be helpful to review with the adoptive parents the child's progress in responding to a more appropriate pattern of emotional responsiveness, in the light of their vulnerabilities and resilience. This can help to highlight any areas of success, even where progress is slow.

We also need to assess

- how far any problems that have arisen relate directly to the child's difficulties, e.g. with developing more secure attachments
- whether they are linked to the capacity of the adoptive parents to provide for the child's specific needs or difficulties
- if they relate to the adoptive parents' own difficulties, e.g. with unresolved losses activated by caring for the child
- how the adoptive parents understand the barriers to responding to the needs of the child.

On the basis of this assessment we can identify the support the parents may need to overcome the barriers.

The *HOME Inventory* (Cox and Walker 2002) specifically addresses emotional sensitivity and responsivity of the caregiver towards the child and helps to locate the exact nature of the difficulties the adoptive parents are experiencing in day-to-day care. The *Family Assessment* (Bentovim and Bingley Miller 2001) helps to assess salient aspects of parenting and in the context of family life such as how feelings are expressed and responded to, whether relationships are supportive and appreciative or rejecting or devaluing, the level of emotional involvement, the nature of attachments and the nature of the parent–child and other alliances.

Case example – respite care for a 14-year-old boy with an attachment disorder

Assessment

John was 14 years old and had lived with his adoptive family for ten years. He was severely neglected and abused in his birth family and was a troubled boy when he was placed for adoption. His adoptive parents had done their best to provide emotional warmth but were aware John had a limited capacity to accept it. School was always a difficult place for him and he had a full statement of special needs for emotional and behavioural difficulties. He was on Ritalin as he had many of the symptoms of ADHD and had also been diagnosed as having an attachment disorder. His adoptive parents had always found him hard work and had attended training days and seminars and used the behaviour strategies they'd learnt to try and help John. However, as he moved into adolescence in his behaviour at home got worse. He was staying out late, drinking and smoking, truanting from school and becoming increasingly verbally and physically abusive towards his adoptive mother. His parents were exhausted, and although they loved their son they knew they needed breaks from the responsibility of caring for him and for the sake of their younger daughter, who was finding it very stressful having John in the house.

Support/intervention

The social services post-adoption specialist offered short breaks for John to give his parents regular weekend breaks to recharge their batteries every other weekend. This has allowed John to remain part of his family, by giving his parents the breaks they need to continue the hard work of parenting him.

As with many attachment-disordered children, John is not prone to physical violence against adults other than his adoptive parent and the specialist adolescent foster carer he goes to manages the respite care quite well. She has an older adopted son and seems to understand both John's needs and the needs of these adoptive parents.

> ## Pointers for practice in emotional warmth
>
> - Emotional warmth is essential for the development of the adopted child's capacity to make supportive social relationships.
> - But there is a range of adopted children, including many of those with disorganised attachment patterns, who may not respond readily, if ever, to the emotional warmth provided by their adoptive parents. Some adoptive parents will need specialist help and support to assess and plan how best to respond to their child's emotional needs.
> - Assessments of the emotional responsiveness of adoptive parents towards the adopted child in the context of the child's earlier experiences of how feelings and emotions were dealt can help gauge the adoption support a child and/or their family may need.
> - An assessment of the current state of the adopted child's attachments may be required to understand the difficulties encountered by adoptive parents and their support needs.
> - Adoptive parents may need specialist help or training to be able to provide the particular pattern of emotional responsiveness required to address the complex needs of some adopted children.
> - The experience of caring for an adopted child can reactivate unresolved emotional issues for adopters and workers need to be able to recognise the presence of such issues and to help adoptive parents to find the support and/or therapeutic help they need to address them.

Stimulation

Stimulation relates to the need to promote a child's learning and intellectual development through encouragement, cognitive stimulation and providing social opportunities. Includes facilitating the child's cognitive development and potential through interaction, communication, talking and responding to the child's language and questions, encouraging and joining the child's play, and promoting educational opportunities. Enabling the child to experience success and ensuring school attendance or equivalent opportunity. Facilitating child to meet the challenges of life.

(DoH et al. 2000b: 21)

It is important that the level of stimulation, encouragement or warmth that adopted children may or may not have received earlier in their lives and how this links to the cognitive development of the child is as well documented as possible so that prospective adoptive parents can be fully briefed prior to placement.

The adoption support component of the Placement Plan will need to assess the new adoptive parents' understanding of the adopted child's needs in this area, plan with them how to provide the stimulation and play or learning opportunities their child will need and to consider any support that is required.

Where there are concerns about the stimulation being provided for an adopted child, it is helpful to assess the adoptive parents' understanding of the child's specific needs in the light of their previous experiences, their level of cognitive development and their age. The assessment may reveal that adoptive parents require help in identifying the pattern of stimulation, encouragement and warmth to help a child overcome barriers presented by the impact of earlier adverse experiences, or to respond to their special needs which are the result of physical impairments or learning difficulties. A referral to a speech and language specialist may be indicated to help the adoptive parents promote the child's communication skills. Assessment may include consideration of the financial support that may be required to enable parents to provide learning and social opportunities for a child.

Several subscales of the *HOME Inventory* (Cox and Walker 2002) cover stimulation, support and opportunities for play and learning provided by the adoptive parents that support the cognitive development of the adopted child. This includes the provision of play and learning materials, language and academic stimulation and encouragement of play and learning. The *Family Activities Scales* identify child-centred family activities and support for independent activity. The *Family Assessment* (Bentovim and Bingley Miller 2001) explores how adoptive parents promote a child's development through stimulation, emotional warmth and praise.

Where the difficulties are severe it can be helpful to take a multi-agency approach at an early stage both to the assessment of the problems and the provision of support that may involve both school or nursery and CAMHS or other specialist services.

Case example – responding to the special care needs of an adopted child with physical disabilities

Assessment

James was a 2-year-old adopted boy with a genetic condition resulting in his feet being turned inwards, loose joints and limited manual dexterity. He needed constant stimulation to strengthen the muscles in his limbs, best done through play and exercises.

Support/intervention

In placement an inter-agency system was set up to teach and guide the adopters in this work which included paediatrician, portage worker, physiotherapist and occupational therapist. The adopters had to be able to work with many professionals, a major requirement in the matching process. Later the adopters wanted James to attend the local playgroup but had to stay with the child because of his special needs. The adoption agency providing post adoption support arranged for a specialist key worker to be trained by the adopters and professionals in stimulating the child's muscle development through play and encouraging his mobility. James could then be left by the adopters just like all the other children.

Pointers for practice in stimulation

- Many adopted children are delayed in their cognitive development and need extra support, encouragement, stimulation and opportunities to learn and develop in order to catch up.
- Parents may need assistance in understanding and supporting the developmental stage of their adopted child taking into account their chronological age and any developmental delay or disability.
- Parents may need help in developing skills in providing the specific stimulation and learning and social opportunities their child needs to promote their development.
- Parents often join the family life cycle rather abruptly and may not have built up relationships with the nursery or school or other families with children. They may value help establishing these links so that their adopted child can take a fuller part in the associated social and educational opportunities.
- Specialist advice and financial support may be required where adoptive parents are caring for an adopted child with more severe emotional problems, learning difficulties and other disabilities.

Guidance and boundaries

Guidance and boundaries includes enabling the child to regulate their own emotions and behaviour. The key parental tasks are demonstrating and modelling appropriate behaviour and control of emotions and interactions with others, and guidance, which involves setting boundaries, so that the child is able to develop a internal model of moral values and conscience, and social behaviour appropriate for the society within which they will grow up. The aim is to enable the child to grow up into an autonomous adult, holding their own values, and able to demonstrate appropriate behaviour with others rather than having to dependent on rules outside themselves. This includes not over protecting children from exploratory and learning experiences. Includes social problem solving, anger management, consideration for others, and effective discipline and shaping of behaviour.

(DoH et al. 2000b: 21)

It is important to understand the specific needs of an adopted child for guidance and boundaries when assessing any problems adoptive parents may be having in this difficult area. Children with emotional and behavioural difficulties often require careful boundary setting and guidance. Those who have, for example, identified with aggressive parental role models or experienced chaotic family and social relationships in their birth family will bring high levels of need and it will be challenging to establish effective and appropriate boundaries, guidance and modelling for them. As part of the assessment for support needs, it is therefore often useful to link back to earlier assessments, which give information about the environments in which the adopted child has previously lived to understand any links with the difficulties the adoptive parents are currently encountering, what may need to change and the support parents may need to achieve this change.

The *HOME Inventory* (Cox and Walker 2002) specifically addresses modelling by parents and the use of boundaries in parent–child relationships, how the parent disciplines the child, how they encourage the development of socially responsible and mature behaviour and how they set limits for children. The *Family Assessment* (Bentovim and Bingley Miller 2001) looks at strengths and difficulties the parents have in providing guidance, boundary setting, protection and their expectations of the children, and associated aspects of family life which affect how the adoptive parents manage guidance and boundaries, including decision making and problem solving and the management of conflicts. The *Parenting Daily Hassles Scale* helps to establish current areas of difficulty or strain adoptive parents may be encountering particularly with managing children's behaviour at home and in public. On the basis of such an assessment it is possible to suggest whether specific parenting skills advice or training or other forms of support may be required to help adoptive parents cope more confidently and establish more positive relationships in the family.

Where there are difficulties with face-to-face contact with birth families, it is sometimes necessary to assess the appropriateness of the guidance and boundaries provided at contact to decide what support is needed to ensure the adopted child's needs are responded appropriately.

Pointers for practice in guidance and boundaries

- Children require guidance and boundaries within a stable family environment if they are to develop into secure, autonomous, independent and responsible adults.
- Many children adopted from the care system have lived in the context of family instability and inconsistent parenting which has affected their capacity to trust others and make new relationships. Parents may need help to set boundaries and provide guidance which supports the emotional and behavioural developmental needs of the child.
- Information about how guidance, care and management of the child and tasks such as decision making and managing conflicts were managed in their birth family can help adoptive parents understand their adopted child's specific needs for guidance and boundaries.
- Information about how adopted children have responded in subsequent placements, if they have received skilled and attuned care, can assist adoptive parents predict the approach to establishing boundaries and providing boundaries their child will need.
- Some adopted children who have experienced significant instability and inconsistent guidance and boundaries respond with aggressive and/or destructive behaviour, causing much distress to their adoptive families who may require specialist help in containing the behaviour and responding to the child's needs.

- Difficulties with face-to-face contact with birth families sometimes relate to the guidance and boundaries provided and an assessment of the support needs for those involved may be required.
- There is evidence that factors which significantly affect the risk of break-down in fostering placements include lack of parental confidence, behaviour in children which their foster carers find problematic and lack of 'click' when carers feel they do not understand a child and can not get on with them. Practice wisdom indicates that these factors are also relevant in adoptive placements.
- There is also evidence that parenting skills programmes, specifically designed to help adoptive parents develop the enhanced parenting skills which their adopted children may require, are effective and support services should include access to such programmes.
- Adopted children may display behaviour at school or nursery which staff find problematic, or have difficulties in their peer relationships. Liaison between the adoptive family and the school (and, if necessary, the local education authority and specialist sources of educational help) may be useful to make sure that 'adoption aware' assessments of the child's needs and plans for intervention are made.

Stability

Stability involves providing a sufficiently stable family environment to enable a child to develop and maintain a secure attachment to the primary caregiver(s) in order to ensure optimal development. Includes ensuring secure attachments are not disrupted, providing consistency of emotional warmth over time and respond-ing in a similar manner to the same behaviour. Parental responses change and develop according to the child's developmental progress. In addition, ensuring children keep in contact with important family members and significant others.

(DoH et al. 2000b: 21)

To assess the support needs of adoptive parents in this area, workers need to have a working understanding of the different patterns of attachment, i.e. secure, inse-cure and disorganised, and how they develop. Because of their background of instability, adopted children often have high levels of need in this area. Workers need to appreciate the challenges to adoptive parents which the associated behav-iour and emotional responses of their adopted children can present.

Information from previous assessments of an adopted child's emotional and behavioural development, especially concerning their attachments, helps to identify the enhanced or 'parenting plus' skills they are likely to require and the support adoptive parents may need to establish a stable environment for the child.

It is important to identify and build on the strengths in adoptive parents' approaches to providing the care their children need and to establish where they are finding difficulties. The *HOME Inventory* (Cox and Walker 2002) provides infor-mation about aspects such as parental responsivity and acceptance and the emotional climate. The *Family Assessment* (Bentovim and Bingley Miller 2001) helps to assess the nature of the attachments and of the parent–child relationship and how feelings are expressed and responded to in the family.

If adoptive parents request support post-placement, it is important to assess how far they have been able to help the adopted child to develop an attachment to them and to provide consistent emotional warmth in response to the child's changing needs. We also need to know, where relevant, how adoptive parents are managing balancing this with facilitating contact with significant members of the child's birth family. Where there are difficulties, sometimes the stability of the adopted child's place in their adoptive family is developing effectively but at the cost of links with the birth relatives or others being less well maintained. Sometimes the difficulties over contact are seriously undermining the stability the adoptive parents are able to offer the child.

It is sometimes necessary to explore and assess how far the adoptive parents are able to talk with the adopted child about their birth family and their place in the adoptive family, as this an area where they may need support.

Case example – balancing needs for maintaining sibling relationships with security of attachment in new family

Assessment

Conflict arose in a pre-adoptive placement where a sibling group of three children had been placed, George, a boy of 9 years, and Lucy and Annie, two younger sisters of 7 and 5 years. The children had been removed from a highly abusive family context and had been placed in foster care where the foster carers had applied to adopt the children but had been rejected. The placement for adoption continued to encompass contact with the previous foster carers with whom there had been a strong alliance formed. Goerge's placement with the prospective adoptive family broke down and he was returned to the former foster family with a request that the two younger children be returned with him to maintain the tie between them and the relationship with the former foster carers, who were perceived as important individuals for all three children. Specialist assessment indicated that the attachment between the two girls and the prospective adoptive parents had grown considerably, and there was a prospect of developing a far more secure attachment. It was also revealed that there had been some sexual behaviour enacted between the brother and sisters that indicated that a sibling placement may not have been in their best interests. It appeared that their relationship mirrored the behaviour in their birth family, which had led to their placement first for fostering, and subsequently for adoption.

Support/intervention

It was felt that with extensive support and therapeutic help the prospective adoptive parents could care for the two girls effectively, and it was in their best interests to remain there while maintaining regular contact with their brother. Some mediation work was also required between the former foster family and the adoptive family to ensure that contact arrangements could be satisfactorily maintained.

Case example – helping a child understand their history

Assessment

Kayleigh was an 11-year-old child who was adopted aged 6 following the murder of her mother by her father. She had supervised contact with her maternal grandmother twice a year. Over a period of six months, Kayleigh has told her teachers and her social worker that she is being ill treated at home and wishes to leave her adoptive family. The allegations Kayleigh made were found to be unsubstantiated. Using the *Family Assessment* 'Mapping the Problem' section helped identify the different perceptions of each family member about the problem and the work required to move ahead (Bentovim and Bingley Miller 2001).

Support/intervention

Over time and with detailed work with the child and support of her adoptive parents, Kayleigh began to understand more of her background and why she could not remain in the care of her natural family. The adoptive parents, with support, met with the maternal grandmother every three months so that better communication was facilitated generally so that Kayleigh did not need to split her two worlds. Using the *Adolescent Wellbeing Scale* it was possible to monitor Kayleigh's increased and improved self-esteem (DoH et al. 2000a).

Pointers for practice in stability

- Parents have the task of providing a stable family environment for adopted children who have experienced instability and disrupted attachments so that they can, if possible, develop more secure attachments.
- Parents are likely to have to work extra hard to help their adopted child build an attachment with them, and some children will never be able to do this.
- Workers need to have an understanding of how attachments develop, how they can be supported and how to access specialist help for adoptive families and children if they have severe or persistent difficulties.
- Parents may need support in understanding their adopted child's attachment difficulties and developing the pattern of parenting and care most likely to help their child settle and make attachments.
- The Placement Plan and the Adoption Support Plan should address the support adoptive parents need to manage the child's transition into their family as smoothly as possible.
- Contact with birth families can impact on the stability of the adoptive family. It is important to assess the support adoptive parents may need in

managing, reviewing and/or changing contact arrangements when the stability of the placement or the adopted child's sense of belonging in the adoptive family is being threatened.

- When adopted children want to know more about their birth family, especially if they want to search for their birth family, the support needs of both child or young person and the adoptive parents should be assessed.
- Other adopted or birth children in adoptive families may need support if an adopted sibling is having difficulties or needing a lot of attention.

Chapter 7

Assessing family and environmental factors using the *Assessment Framework*

This chapter addresses the family and environmental factors which can come into play for adoptive and birth families and which may affect an adopted child's developmental needs directly or impact upon the capacity of the adoptive parents to care for the child.

> *The care and upbringing of children does not take place in a vacuum. All family members are influenced both positively and negatively by the wider family, the neighbourhood and social networks in which they live. The history of the child's family and of the individual family members may have a significant impact on the child and parents. A range of environmental factors can either help or hinder a family's functioning.*
>
> (DoH et al. 2000b: 22)

The factors in the family and environmental domain provide the environment within which the adopted child and family live and they are central to the child's well-being and development and the adoptive parents' ability to provide effective parenting.

Adoptive families and special guardians may need help from support services in any one of these areas. Workers should work in partnership with families to provide or help them to access support. This may include liaising with the relevant agencies, or supporting families in obtaining services.

All parents have a similar need to feel valued and supported, especially those caring for children who have come to adoption through the looked after system. It is essential that adoptive families are supported in maintaining the strengths in their family life and the relationships that help them to care effectively for the children and that they receive support and help for any difficulties they may encounter.

Parents therefore benefit from professionals who respect and value their strengths and the major contribution they are making in offering a life-chance to children, with the hope of promoting their children's wellbeing and development. Parents value professionals for whom the adopted child or young person's bests interests are central and who recognise some of the family or environmental factors which may support or impede them as adoptive parents.

Family history and family functioning

Family history includes both genetic and psychosocial factors. Family functioning is influenced by who is living in the household and how they are related to the child; significant changes in family/household composition; history of childhood experiences of parents; chronology of significant life events and their meaning to family members; nature of family functioning, including sibling relationships and its impact on the child; parental strengths and difficulties, including those of an absent parent; the relationship between separated parents.

(DoH et al. 2000b: 23)

Family history and family functioning create part of the framework within which adopted children are cared for. In terms of family history, adopted children have the challenge of having a birth family with whom they are not living and yet with whom they have a history, as well as an adoptive family with whom they develop a history.

Adoptive parents have the task of helping their adopted child gain a sense of belonging. They have to adapt family functioning to accommodate the needs of their adopted child, which are likely to be greatly influenced by their past experience or history, while continuing to meet the needs of other family members.

With the increase in placements for adoption of older children, and the close association with the birth family that often applies under special guardianship arrangements, there can be complex interrelationships between the child's birth family history and functioning and the impact this may have on the relationships in their current families.

Family history of adoptive family

Adoptive parenting is very different from parenting birth children. Clearly one of the crucial differences is that they are parenting a child who brings with them a past history that can provoke associations and feelings for the adoptive parents themselves and affect the way they experience caring for the adopted child. When this occurs, it is important to assess with parents the relationship between any relevant significant past experiences they have had, and the current difficulties they are encountering.

Loss is a common theme for adopted children, adoptive families and birth families; it will form part of every adoption. Adoptive parents who have not been able to have their own children, for example, may find that living with a child who is not their own, and who is having to cope with his or her own losses, reawakens unresolved feelings concerning their own history. This can make it harder to empathise with their adopted child (Brodzinsky 1987; Harris 2005; Howe 1998).

Therefore, if an adopted child's acute experience of loss has brought up feelings of loss and grief for the adoptive parents, it is important to assess how this is affecting their relationship with the child and what support would help to resolve the difficulties.

There are special issues to consider when working with black families. Many black and minority ethnic adoptive families have experiences of transition and loss and multiple parenting that they have negotiated successfully. Their adaptability and resilience are strengths to be acknowledged and valued that are transferable to the adoption context. Alternatively, the feelings of loss associated with migration, for example, may affect their capacity to parent their adopted children (Duck 2003).

The relationship between birth children of adoptive parents and adopted children can be complex particularly because, as the child grows, they may become increasingly aware of the differences in their histories and their way of becoming part of the family and experience painful feelings about those differences which are a part of daily existence. It is important to cover this in the Home Study, and later, if necessary, to offer support to any birth children in the adoptive family as needed.

The family history component of the *Family Assessment* provides a useful way of systematically exploring past significant events, circumstances and relationships and their meaning for the person involved (Bentovim and Bingley Miller 2001). This can help track and identify unresolved issues from the past which adoptive parents may want help to resolve. The *Adult Wellbeing Scale* looks at how an adult is feeling in terms of depression, anxiety and irritability and can indicate when professional help may be beneficial (DoH et al. 2000a; Snaith et al. 1978). The *Recent Life Events Questionnaire* can be very helpful in identifying events that may have put extra strain on adoptive parents (Brugha et al. 1985; DoH et al. 2000a). The *Alcohol Use Questionnaire* can provide a useful starting point for a discussion of any potential difficulties with alcohol use (DoH et al. 2000a; Piccinelli et al. 1997).

Case example – managing losses for an adopted child and adoptive parents

Gemma, Leah and Gordon were a group of two sisters and a brother now aged 12, 10 and 8 years who were placed with a childless couple after being abandoned by their mother three years before. She has never been traced. The children had been well cared for until their mother's departure, which distressed them very much. Considerable work was undertaken in helping the children and the placement was successful until the adoptive mother's own parents died one after the other. The youngest child, Gordon, started to soil himself and also refused to attend school. The *Family Assessment* was used to help the whole family to look at the nature of the children's attachments and to work with the adoptive parents alone on aspects of family history. This helped to reveal their distress at not being able to provide their own parents with birth children and the grief of their infertility and emptiness appeared to have resurfaced. This was also the case for Gordon who needed therapeutic support to help him to understand in a new age appropriate way the loss of his mother.

Family functioning of adoptive families

When adoptive family relationships become affected, it is essential to work collaboratively with the family to identify and understand which areas of family life are currently being affected, and in what ways, so that a plan for providing support can be identified.

Sometimes adoptive families ask for support because they have run into difficulties in family relationships. Children may be fighting and arguing, parent–child relationships may be stressed or marked by arguments or difficulties in communicating. Adults may be having a hard time in their couple relationship or in their parental partnership. Parents who are parenting on their own may feel overwhelmed or in need of support in the face of adopted children who are challenging or distressed.

There is evidence that hurt children, who import the experience of troubled and distorted family relationships, find the vulnerable aspects of their parents as people or of their relationship and expose those vulnerabilities. They do this in ways that the adoptive parents would be unlikely to face with children who had not had those damaging early experiences in their birth families (Steele et al. 2003).

In these circumstances, assessing how families are currently functioning forms a crucial part of any assessment of adoption support needs. To plan effective support, it is important to discriminate between difficulties in family relationships that arise from the adoptive family's own existing difficulties, and those difficulties which relate to disturbed, distressing or disruptive patterns of relating imported by an adopted child from their birth family.

Assessment should also identify family strengths that can be built upon as well as looking at areas of difficulty and how they can best be addressed. The original assessment of the adoptive parents as prospective adopters can be a very useful basis for looking at the family strengths, skills and competencies that can be built upon when planning what support the family may feel they need. The assessment may have also identified areas of potential vulnerability that the adopters may need help with if a child present difficulties.

When assessing adopters it is important to get a sense of the stability of their relationship, their attachments and their support systems to understand how they are likely to respond to some of the pressures of adoption. The *Attachment Style Interview* helps to identify the attachment style of prospective adopters, how they relate to their partner and/or very close others, and their attitudes towards relationships with other people and how they use their support systems (Bifulco et al. 2002a, 2002b). This can be very helpful in planning what support adoptive parents may need at times of stress.

Crucial everyday interactions and operations of family life may need to be understood to plan effective support, for example, decision making, problem solving, managing and resolving conflict, the characteristic way people communicate, how feelings are expressed and responded to, the nature of the different relationships in the family and how issues of identity are handled. The *Family Assessment* provides a systematic and evidence-based approach to assessing family life and relationships and can be adapted for use with adoptive families.

Case example – working with family strengths

Assessment

James, who is 9 years old, came into care at 3 years old following a non-accidental injury to his skull while in the care of his parents and had also been exposed to neglect and emotional abuse. He was placed with foster carers as a short-term measure where his behaviour was oppositional and chaotic. He was aggressive and often placed himself in dangerous situations. The contested legal proceedings took three years to conclude; meanwhile James thrived in his foster placement and his carers were successful in providing security, boundaries and routine. The family wished to adopt James but he had developed serious head pain and became blind in one eye, thought to be as a result of his early skull injury. The family found his increasing dependency very difficult to manage and their own young teenage daughter began to act out and started to run away from home. Use of the *Family Assessment* (Bentovim and Bingley Miller 2001) helped the family and worker to trace their strengths in being able to all pull together in difficult situations, but identified that they needed help in addressing and coming to terms with their daughter's autonomy as well as some gender differences in parenting which sometimes compounded the difficulties.

Support/intervention

Helping the family to realise their strengths and identify the successes enabled them to tackle the future, which included the adoption of James.

Pointers for practice in family history and family functioning

- Children who are adopted or cared for by special guardians have the challenge of having a birth family with which they have a history and becoming a permanent member of an adoptive family. Parents have the challenge of adapting their functioning to accommodate to the needs of their adopted child.
- Preparation and assessment of adopters should include exploration of their own history of attachment, loss, abuse or trauma and their responses, in order to identify where they may need support or help, if caring for a troubled adopted child reactivates unresolved issues in a way which affects their relationship with the child.
- Parents need to be supported and valued in maintaining their family life and relationships and given access to support if they run into difficulties.
- Adoptive family members may need help to explore troubling issues from their own past history if these surface as a result of aspects of caring for their adopted child.

- The adaptability and resilience of many black families in response to adverse life experiences and the impact of discrimination and racism should both be recognised and valued when planning adoption support.
- Difficulties in adoptive family functioning may result from the impact of disturbed patterns of relating imported by the adopted child from earlier relationships they have experienced, or they may relate to existing issues in the adoptive family.
- Understanding the adopted child's past experiences and the family history and family functioning of the adoptive family helps to identify strengths on which they can draw and any areas of vulnerability for which they may need support.
- Adopted children and families may need specialist help to resolve family relationship difficulties. It is crucial that professionals offering support or therapeutic help are 'adoption aware' and can understand and discriminate between the considerable impact on family relationships a troubled adopted child can bring and any difficulties the adoptive family may already have.
- There are many forms of adoption support that families may appreciate when their family life or relationships are under pressure, ranging from practical help through to special therapeutic help or counselling.

Wider family

Who are considered to be members of the wider family by the child and parents? Includes related and non-related person and absent wider family. What is their role and importance to child and parents and in precisely what way?

(DoH et al. 2000b: 23)

The wider adoptive family

Contact with the child's wider adoptive family can be a rich and rewarding experience for adopted children, and give them a sense of belonging and acceptance within a wider family. Any assessment of adoption support needs should include consideration of whether the wider family need support to maximise their positive involvement with the adopted child, and for them to be able to provide support for the adoptive parents.

Where there are difficulties in relationships with the wider adoptive family, it may be helpful to find out whether it is hard for significant family members to understand the extra care needs of adopted children and the special challenges involved in parenting them. Some children displaying attachment disordered behaviour present this in a range of social situations. Others exhibit aggressive or rejecting behaviour only towards their adoptive parents. This creates difficulties especially for new adoptive parents who may become exhausted but feel their wider family do not understand. Relatives of adoptive parents are not usually including in the training and process of preparation for the match and yet they may be a major source of potential support.

Adoptive grandparents, aunts and uncles may find the behaviour of the adopted child or the difficulties faced by the adoptive parents in caring for the child puzzling and may be critical of the approach being taken by the adoptive parents. They may not understand a child's attachment difficulties, for example, and begin to question the parents' capabilities when the child takes a long time to settle, or 'misbehaves'. This can lead to arguments or a withdrawal of valuable support and a potential loss for the adopted child.

Alternatively, some adoptive family relatives may actually find playing their part in taking care of the adopted child too hard in the way they might expect to as relatives, given the child's special needs. This can be disappointing for adoptive parents and lead to family difficulties. An assessment of their views and difficulties in relating to the adopted child, or understanding their needs, can help identify the support that would help resolve some of these issues.

For white adoptive families who have adopted a black child, there may be issues that need assessing about how the child is accepted by the wider family and with which the child and adoptive parents may need support.

Friendships and faith communities

Close friends are often a significant source of support to adoptive parents and if there have been any difficulties in maintaining adoptive parents' support networks, it is important to assessment the nature of the difficulties to see whether they can be supported. Sometimes friends, like relations, need information and advice about the special challenges of adoption and adoptive parenting. Similarly faith communities provide spiritual, emotional and practical support. Sometimes the demands of adoptive parenting and the needs of adopted children can present lead to difficulties in accessing the support of the faith community in a similar way.

The adopted child's wider family – contact with the child's immediate birth family

When assessing the support needs of those involved in contact, it is important to have a clear idea of the purpose of the contact, i.e. which particular needs of the adopted child is it intended to meet (Neil 2002). The quality of contact can then be defined in terms of the extent to which it helps child meet these needs. Contact with birth relatives should then be considered in terms of what potential the birth family has to assist the child with his/her individual needs, as above. When adoptive parents seek help with contact, a careful assessment should be made of the nature and management of contact and the support needs of all concerned and a support plan drawn up on the basis of those needs.

It is important to note that the assessment of the impact of contact on the adopted child's emotional wellbeing is a central element in assessing support needs. From the adopted child's perspective it may be important to distinguish between different birth relatives as high priority often needs to be given to maintaining contact between brothers and sisters who have lived together. Contact with grandparents, uncles and aunts, previous foster carers who have been significant and not identified with abuse or abusing parents can be especially important.

Families from different cultural and ethnic backgrounds have different ways of defining family members and it is important to establish which significant adults are seen as members of the wider family network so that an accurate assessment of support needs can be made (Charlton et al. 1998; Harris 2005).

When there are difficulties with contact, this can impact on the adopted child's wellbeing and their behaviour within the adoptive family. Further assessment may be required to provide the basis for planning, if possible alongside the birth family, how contact can be supported and managed in a way that reduces the pressures on the child. Where contact continues to have a negative impact on the adopted child's wellbeing, assessment may indicate that it should cease.

Case example – contact and children who feel responsible for birth parents

Assessment

Jill, Hannah and Rick aged 16, 15 and 13 were placed with a foster family three years previously and remained in monthly contact with their birth parents, who had learning difficulties. The children worried about their parents and were anxious when they enjoyed themselves as they felt they should be at home looking after their parents. Hannah, the middle child, expressed feelings of divided loyalties and spoke of distressing memories of the past. She then became anorexic and the whole family struggled to cope. Jill, the eldest child, dominated her sister and sometimes it was hard for Hannah to say what she really felt. Mapping the current concerns and difficulties with the family, using the *Family Assessment* (Bentovim and Bingley Miller 2001), helped to clarify how each person saw the problem and looking at family alliances enabled the foster parents to examine and adapt how they interacted within the family.

Support/intervention

Further individual work with each of the children was indicated to help them relinquish their sense of responsibility for their birth parents.

An important consideration in assessing contact needs will be the adopted child's wishes and feelings. Research studies of adopted children demonstrate that generally children want to keep in touch with birth relatives and feel unhappy when they lose contact (Macaskill 2002; Thomas et al. 1999). However, children do discriminate between different relatives and may wish to cease contact with certain relatives, especially when the person concerned has been rejecting or hostile.

For birth relatives whose child is placed for adoption, adjusting to the loss of their child and the related changes in their role, is an additional psychological task which is naturally very challenging and with which they may need help for themselves in their own right. It is also the case that birth relatives are most likely to be a resource to a child in their new family if they can accept and support the child's placement and work collaboratively with adoptive parents. The success or otherwise of birth relatives in making these adjustments is likely to be relevant to the child's future wellbeing, particularly in relation to contact.

It is therefore important to assess the support needs that birth relatives may have and the services or resources that could help them to adjust to their child's adoption or move to be cared for by special guardians. This may involve working with them to understand the significant issues for them that relate to the process and experience of their child being adopted and what support they might find most helpful.

Birth parents in contact with their adopted children should have their own assessment of support needs and their own worker. Birth relatives may need support in managing or maintaining contact meetings or sending letters. There is considerable research evidence to suggest that sustaining quality contact with adopted children and looked after children can be very difficult for birth relatives because of practical and emotional barriers (Masson et al. 1997; Milham et al. 1986).

Assessments should take into account these barriers and offer the services or resources to help remove them. This relates back to the purpose of contact for adopted children. If good quality contact is thought of as a resource to the adopted child, then barriers to the achievement and maintenance of such contact need to be removed, not erected.

Face-to-face contact

In many cases where adopted children have established relationships with birth relatives, however, such attachments may be insecure and the child may have experienced poor care or maltreatment within these relationships. Past difficulties may continue to be evident in contact meetings and the child can be left with a mixture of feelings that show themselves as difficult behaviours.

Sometimes birth family members continue to demonstrate during contact the same behaviours that had led to the child's admission to care, for example, unpredictable or entangled relationships being played out in contact visits (Schofield et al. 2000). Contact in these circumstances will inevitably be a complex experience for the child, and in the event of difficulties the value of contact should be carefully reassessed and may need to be stopped, particularly if it threatens the stability of the adoptive placement.

There are a range of ways of assessing the meaning and impact of contact on the adopted child and the adoptive family. The *HOME Inventory* (Cox and Walker 2002) often helps to understand how contact may be affecting how the child reacts in their adoptive family. *In My Shoes* (Calam et al. 2000) provides a non-threatening way to explore a child's feelings about the dilemmas and emotions they may be faced with regarding contact. The *Adolescent Wellbeing Scale* or the *Strengths and Difficulties Questionnaire* (DoH et al. 2000a) may help identify the impact in terms of the child's emotional and behavioural wellbeing and development. The

Family Assessment (Bentovim and Bingley Miller 2001) can help identify both strengths and vulnerabilities in the way contact issues impact on adoptive family relationships.

Case example – ensuring appropriate contact with a birth mother

Assessment

Susie, an infant, was placed by her mother for fostering with a view to considering adoption because she was diagnosed with AIDS during the pregnancy and because of experiences in her country of origin feared that she would not recover. Susie was placed in a carefully culturally matched context, and there was an agreement that there would be continuing contact, which in the early months was well maintained. The foster mother, although initially considered a short-term bridging placement while long-term planning was considered, applied to adopt herself. There was an agreement that this was an appropriate placement for the child and contact with the birth mother continued. Because of a change in her circumstances, regular contact lessened in frequency, and the good relationship established between the birth mother and the prospective adoptive mother deteriorated. The prospective adoptive mother was concerned that, because of an improvement in the birth mother's state, she might wish to claim the child back in line with her cultural beliefs shared by both mother and prospective adopters. The prospective adoptive mother's care deteriorated, she became depressed, it became evident that she had not wished to inform Susie adequately about the nature of her birth, and the relationship between herself and the birth mother. There was concern that this was emotionally abusive to the child. The appropriateness of the placement was reviewed, given that the birth mother wanted the child returned to her care and her health was now improving. It became evident on specialist assessment that the attachment between the child and prospective adoptive mother was now firmly established, and in general terms she was making good progress in all areas and had some well-formed ideas about who was who in her life.

Support/intervention

With confirmation of the child's best interests, mediation work between the adoptive mother and the birth mother continued and it became possible to plan an appropriate supportive approach to ensuring that Susie was given appropriate knowledge of her parentage, and why adoption was felt to be in her interests. The connection between adoptive and birth mother was re-established in a way which met the child's needs.

Contact between adopted child and their birth brothers and sisters

Contact with birth brothers and sisters can be very important for adopted children and may need to be prioritised. There is a crucial role for workers in assessing the support needs of adoptive families and children, and birth families if they are involved, to help them maintain and change contact arrangements between brothers and sisters. The support needed may be financial, practical, advice or information, helping families exchange information or offering a base for reviewing contact and planning changes or mediating any difficulties.

Pointers for practice in the wider family

- The wider adoptive family can help to develop an adopted child's sense of belonging, being appreciated and valued as a family member and increase their skills in social relationships.
- Sometimes members of the wider adoptive family, including grandparents, are unsupportive towards adoptive parents because they do not understand the special needs of adopted children. This reduces the support network for adoptive parents and the richness of being accepted into a wider family network for the adopted child.
- The wider adoptive family need access to support services. Preparation and training of wider adoptive family members can be helpful.
- Continuity and contact with their birth family can be very beneficial for an adopted child. Most contact is indirect, with only a small proportion of adopted children having face-to-face contact with birth relatives. All contact plans must be clear about the purpose of contact, the arrangements and take into account the wishes and feelings of the child and adoptive parents.
- Contact plans work best when both adoptive parents and birth relatives are motivated to maintain contact for an adopted child and have agreed when and how contact will take place. Both families may need support in working out plans that benefit the child the most and cause the least pressure for all concerned.
- Contact can be one of the more stressful aspects of adoption for children, adoptive families and birth families and may at times, risk the stability of a placement.
- Parents and adopted children may seek support with adjusting or changing contact plans when the child's needs change over time or the contact presents difficulties for an adopted child or either family.
- ASSAs and other workers have a key role in assessing changing support needs. Mediation and negotiation may be required to reach agreement over new contact plans. Birth relatives may need support in maintaining or relinquishing contact if there is a change of plan.
- Services that provide staffed and, where necessary, properly supervised locations for contact are an important part of adoption services.

> - It may help adopted children to settle in their adoptive family if they have contact with significant attachment figures from their birth family, such as grandparents, or previous substitute families.
> - The role of other significant adults from the wider family in the life of the child prior to placement should be assessed so that contact can be planned in the best interests of the child.

Housing

Does accommodation have basic amenities and facilities appropriate to the age and development of the child and other resident members? Is the housing accessible and suitable to the needs of disabled family members? Includes the interior and exterior of the accommodation and immediate surroundings. Basic amenities include water, heating, sanitation, cooking facilities, sleeping arrangements and cleanliness, hygiene and safety and their impact on the child's upbringing.

(DoH et al. 2000b: 23)

Housing is an important part of the environment when caring for an adopted child. The housing needs of adoptive families are often different from other families. Adoptive families will have been assessed as having adequate housing, but they may need financial assistance or help with liasing with housing authorities to be able to access housing suitable for the specific needs of the children for whom they are caring.

It is important to ensure there is sufficient space for all the children when an adopted child joins a family. This is particularly so where a large group of brothers and sisters are placed together, or where potential difficulties in the relationship between adopted brothers and sisters have been identified. Not many families can take a large sibling group without extending their present home, and housing needs will have to be kept under review as the children grow.

It is important, however, to recognise and respect cultural differences where appropriate. For example, in many Punjabi families, brothers and sisters sharing a bedroom is seen as desirable and such customary practices should be taken into account when assessing support needs.

The way the special care needs of some adopted children relates to housing sometimes requires careful assessment for support needs. Children who have been sexually abused should not usually have to share a room at any age and for some it may be important that alarms on bedroom doors are fitted so that children cannot move from room to room undetected.

Other adopted children may have special needs regarding space because they have mobility impairments. The ASSA should be able to broker appropriate arrangements with the local housing authority to provide adapted housing to support the placement.

The *HOME Inventory* (Cox and Walker 2002) provides information on housing as part of an assessment of the adopted child's home environment. The *Recent Life Events Questionnaire* (DoH et al. 2000a) helps to assess the impact of recent house moves, which can be a major life event for family members. Both can therefore be helpful in identify support needs and planning the services or support that may be required. The *Home Conditions Scale* addresses standards of cleanliness (Davie et al. 1984; DoH et al. 2000a).

Pointers for practice in housing

- Adoptive families may need financial assistance or help with liaising with housing authorities to be able to access housing suitable for the specific needs of the children they are caring for. They should also have access to financial advice as part of their Adoption Support Plan where appropriate.
- Housing may need to be extended or adapted to accommodate the needs of a large sibling groups, or adopted children who need their own bedroom.
- Adopted disabled children, in particular, may need special housing or adaptations to existing housing.
- ASSAs can play a coordinating role between the adoptive family and relevant professionals to make sure that their housing can meet the needs of their adopted child.

Employment

Who is working in the household, their pattern of work and any changes? What impact does this have on the child? How is work or absence of work viewed by family members? How does it affect their relationship with the child? Includes children's experience of work and its impact on them.

(DoH et al. 2000b: 23)

Children who are adopted or cared for by special guardians often need more time and attention and enhanced parenting skills than other children because they have emotional difficulties or impairments or learning disabilities. This can have an impact on the work patterns of adoptive parents and may mean that one or other parents is unable to work.

It is part of the process of assessing support needs for the Placement Plan to prepare adoptive parents to be aware of the possible impact of the adopted child's ongoing needs on their employment. Parents therefore have to have enough information about a child's needs to be able to be realistic about how their work patterns may affect their capacity to meet those needs. If changes are required, they may need support in achieving these.

Some adoptive parents matched with an adopted child with considerable emotional needs, for example, have the hope and expectation that after a settling-in period they will both be able to return to full-time work. This is clearly sometimes possible for some adopted children and not for others, if their extra care needs are to be optimally met. It is very difficult to predict how long a child will take to settle and it is wise to prepare adoptive parents for the possibility of one of them needing to be away from work for much longer than they have anticipated.

To predict the levels of care an adopted child is likely to need, it is useful if a *HOME Inventory* (Cox and Walker 2002) has been carried out with a birth parent or a foster carer to provide a systematic and detailed picture of the care a child needs and the challenges they may present. This can then help workers, and prospective parents decide whether their employment patterns fit with the needs of the child.

Unexpected difficulties may arise, requiring an assessment of how adoptive parents can be supported over employment issues. Adopted children may not adjust readily to ordinary nursery care, child-minders, after school clubs or holiday schemes. Staff may not be equipped to handle their special care needs or the child may need much more structured and nurturing care than is provided. An extended period of care by one or other parent may be required until the child has become secure enough to be able to handle care by others.

Pointers for practice in employment

- It is important that in the preparation for matching, adoptive parents are given a realistic picture of how the adopted child's care needs may impact on their employment pattern.
- Adopted children's care needs can change and adoptive parents may need financial help or advice if one has to give up work unexpectedly because of their child's needs.
- Adoptive parents should have access to information that helps them make the best use of statutory leave and pay arrangements and other allowances and benefits; this is part of an adoption support service.

Income

Income available over a sustained period of time. Is the family in receipt of all its benefit entitlements? Sufficiency of income to meet the family's needs. The way resources available to family are used. Are there financial difficulties which affect the child.

(DoH et al. 2000b: 23)

The Adoption Support Services Guidance states that 'financial barriers should not be the sole reason for adoption failing to go ahead, or to survive' (DoH 2005a) and the Adoption and Children Act 2002 provides for greater flexibility about when financial support can be provided, including post-placement provision.

Caring for adopted children usually demands increased resources to meet their additional needs. It is well recognised that it can cost up to three times more to raise child with disabilities than a child without disabilities (Argent 2003a). These costs need to be taken into account when assessing the adoptive family's financial support needs and ensuring that the child has all the aids and adaptations to which they are entitled. An emotionally needy adopted child may drain parental energy so that help is needed with housework etc. Some forms of emotional disturbance, such as bed wetting, soiling and destructive behaviour, are very costly. Additional therapy or counselling may have to be paid for and extra activities and interests may be important ways of building resilience. An incoming adopted child may detract from the time and resources available to other children in the family and this should be taken into account. At the very least there will new costs for the family due to the basic upkeep of the child.

At the same time, the family income may be reduced due to one partner doing less or no paid work in order to care adequately for the child. This may impact not only on the family income but also on the career plans and prospects of that parent. In addition, the child's needs might increase over time, necessitating one or both parents to be more available to the child and therefore less available for work. Kinship carers, such as grandparents, have been shown to be reluctant to ask for help and to value clear, written entitlements to levels of support from agencies (Pitcher 2002).

It may be helpful to consider all increased expenditure for the family that is related to the arrival of a new adoptive child within this Income section, pulling together financial implications which have become apparent in other dimensions.

There are certain considerations that local authorities must make when looking at the payment of financial support. These are listed in Regulations 8 and 15 of the Adoption Support Services Regulations 2005. Financial support can be paid only

- where it is necessary to ensure that the adoptive parent can look after the child
- to meet the child's special needs arising from illness, disability or the consequences of past abuse or neglect
- to meet the child's particular needs arising from age or ethnic origin
- to enable siblings to be placed together
- to cover the costs of contact with the birth family or siblings
- to meet the adopters' legal costs
- to meet the cost of introductions
- expenditure necessary for the purpose of accommodating the child, including the provision of furniture and domestic equipment, alterations to and adaptations of the home, provision of means of transport and provision of clothing, toys and other items necessary for the purpose of looking after the child.

It is important at this stage in that process that any benefits, tax credits and other forms of income to which the new adoptive family will be entitled are identified. This is because financial payments made by local authorities to support adoption and special guardianship cannot duplicate those payable under the tax and benefit system. Adoptive parents often need clear advice and guidance from a specialist welfare rights adviser to ensure their benefits are maximised, and the ASSA should be placed to help secure this advice.

Pointers for practice in income

- Caring for adopted children usually involves extra costs and the Adoption and Children Act 2002 Guidance for Children's Services states that 'financial barriers should not be the sole reason for adoption failing to go ahead, or to survive'.

- Assessment of support needs therefore should include, where relevant, an assessment of the financial needs of the adoptive family to enable them to care effectively for their adopted child, as well as coordination between the local authority and adoption agency concerned to ensure that the family receives the financial assistance to which they are entitled.
- Adopted children with special needs such as disabled children and their families may be entitled to special benefits and adoptive parents should be given any information and advice they may need to access those resources. All entitlements to tax credits and benefits in respect of the adoptive family should be established.

Family's social integration

Exploration of the wider context of the local neighbourhood and community and its impact on the child and parents. Includes the degree of the family's integration or isolation, their peer groups, friendship and social networks and the importance attached to them.

(DoH et al. 2000b: 23)

The support network that adoptive families have at the time of placement can become seriously eroded in time as a result of the difficulties the adopted child brings into the family. These families can end up being very socially isolated and any support package should address this. When the degree of social integration or isolation of an adoptive family is being affected by adoption issues it is important to assess what support might be of help for them.

It is a characteristic of adopted children and young people who grow up in families where they have been subject to extensive abuse, rejection or inadequate care, that they may be isolated and not able to integrate easily into their social context, and adoptive families may need support in helping to overcome the barriers to their adopted child being able to join in activities and find peer groups.

Similarly, some adopted children have poor social skills and previous experiences of being rejected by their peers, because of their poor standards of care, hygiene, or clothing. The children may have become involved with the care system and, sadly, this can result in further social isolation; adoptive parents may need support in helping them develop their social skills in social presentation.

Some adopted children may also have had experiences of racism, or heterosexism, or prejudice because they are disabled. The children may therefore have developed defensive strategies that may result in a degree of coping, but at the expense of social integration and may need support with managing experiences of discrimination differently.

Adopted children who have a different racial or cultural background from either their adoptive family and/or the community in which they live may face barriers to their social integration. Workers will need to assess whether adopted children or their families need a referral to an agency which is sensitive to their particular cultural, linguistic or ethnic support needs. They also may need access to information about relevant local minority ethnic communities and resources or activities for black or minority ethnic children and young people. They or their adopted children may need support in helping to manage and counter the experience of racism and discrimination.

Later down the line adoptive parents may feel marginalised because their adopted children are not achieving at school or developing strong friendship groups in the same way as friends' children. Their children may not have the same future plans and may take much longer to leave home. These are also times when adoptive parents may need extra support.

The *Family Activity Scales* (DoH et al. 2000a) and the section in the *Family Assessment* (Bentovim and Bingley Miller 2001) on the family's relationships with the wider family and community can both help to give a picture of the family's relationships with the wider family and the community in which they live and any difficulties they are encountering, including whether the adoptive parents have been able to maintain their friendships.

Pointers for practice in family's social integration

- Adopted children who have experienced serious neglect, abuse, rejection or inadequate care may often lack the skills to integrate socially and become isolated. Children may encounter difficulties in school or nursery or with their peers or others and may experience rejection or bullying.
- Liaison between adoptive parents and school or nursery staff is often important to develop a coherent plan for helping an adopted child to integrate more successfully and to counter problems such as bullying.
- Adoptive parents of children who have a different racial or cultural background from them, or the community in which they live, may need access to information about relevant local minority ethnic communities and resources or activities for black or minority ethnic children and young people. They or their adopted children may need support in helping to manage and counter the experience of racism and discrimination.
- Adoptive parents of minority ethnic backgrounds may need help to access relevant information and services that are sensitive to their ethnic, cultural and linguistic needs.
- New adopters who have not had children of their own can feel marginalised and different and may need help making contact with other families with children of the same age in their community and to locate support groups and training with other adoptive parents.

Community resources

Describes all facilities and services in a neighbourhood, including universal services of primary health care, day care and schools, places of worship, transport, shops and leisure activities. Includes availability, accessibility and standard of resources and impact on family, including disabled members.

(DoH et al. 2000b: 23)

More children are being adopted at a later stage and their needs are often more complex than those of younger children. An extensive range of community resources are required to support adoptive parents and special guardians to help the children achieve their full potential.

Adoptive parents have to be able to access and assess community resources on behalf of their adopted child. An assessment of difficulties they are having in these areas may reveal that they need support in being able to gain information, make contact, advocate for their child for services or overcome barriers to access which may exist.

Providing the right resources requires an assessment of the needs of adopted children resulting from any earlier adverse experiences and the support needs of the adoptive family or special guardian taking on the permanent care of a child. This is particularly important when a child has specific care needs either due to health issues, impairment or learning disability or because they have experienced abuse, rejection and failure of care, separations or losses or trauma, including for example, some children seeking asylum.

Pointers for practice in community resources

- More children are being adopted at a later stage and their needs are often more complex than those of younger children.
- Extensive multi-agency community resources are required to support adoptive parents to help the adopted children they care for achieve their full potential.
- Careful assessment and a thorough knowledge of the local community resources available are needed to match the support needs of adopted children and families with the appropriate community resources.
- Careful and skilled assessment is particularly important when adopted children have special needs for example as a result of physical, sensory or intellectual impairment, inter-country adoption or special health care needs.
- An effective adoption support service needs to have access to an integrated network of social care, education and health services working in a coordinated and collaborative way.
- Managers of support services have a responsibility to plan in partnership with other agencies to ensure that universal, targeted and specialist services are equipped and sufficiently coordinated to be able to respond to the needs of adopted children and children who are cared for by special guardians and their families.

Chapter 8

Responding to needs

Analysing information about needs as the basis for planning support

Planning support for adopted children and their families should be based on a careful analysis of the information which has been collected about child's current developmental needs, the capacity of the adoptive parents to respond to those needs, the impact of any relevant family and environmental factors on the child's needs and on the parenting capacity of the adoptive parents. On the basis of this analysis the worker can make an assessment of the interrelated needs of the adopted child and family. Using this assessment, the worker can then identify the support or interventions to recommend for the adopted child and/or the adoptive family (and the birth family where appropriate) to help meet the child's needs. The DfES *Practice Guidance* on assessing adopters and on assessing support needs of adoptive families provides indicators abut the areas to be addressed in relation to planning adoption support.

Prior to placement: analysing information about needs as a basis for planning support

Prior to placement, in coming to a recommendation about the support or interventions which would assist an adopted child, their prospective adoptive parents and, where appropriate, their birth relatives, it is important to

- draw on assessments which compare the adopted child's responses to parenting in their birth family and in foster care and, in particular, if they have responded to improved parenting capacity
- predict as far as possible what special needs the adopted child is likely to have when placed, including needs for support services
- predict the support the new adoptive parents are likely to require, and whether specific interventions or resources will be needed to develop their parenting capacities to meet the needs of the child
- ascertain whether the new adoptive parents will need support in liaising with other services, for example, education or leisure to ensure the adopted child's needs are responded to appropriately

- ascertain what support members of the birth family may need, especially in relation to maintaining appropriate contact with the child
- be clear about the extent to which needs can be met by the adoption and special guardianship support services which the local authority is required to make arrangements for, or whether wider services from other providers are required.

If this is the case, ensure that there is a coordinated, inter-agency approach to service provision if there is more than one agency likely to be involved with the child

Analysing information about needs as a basis for planning support – post-placement

At the post-placement stage, any assessment process should be attentive to the adoptive parents' views and understanding of the adopted child's difficulties. It should focus on the areas that the adoptive parents (and the child) have identified as problematic, the exact nature of the presenting problem and the underlying needs, the current responses of the adoptive parents and the child, what is working or not working and the impact on the child and the family as a whole. The assessment will also need to take into account the parents' strengths and difficulties in their capacity to meet the needs of the adopted child. The impact of relevant family and environmental factors on adopted child's needs and adoptive parenting capacity also need to be understood before drawing together a plan for support. Workers who have had little experience of working in the field of adoption are likely to need to consult with their AASA when making an assessment and planning support.

It is useful to consider adoptive parenting capacity in the light of the adoptive child's history and their current pattern of vulnerabilities and resilience of the child and to assess

- the adoptive parents' understanding of the adopted child's needs
- the ways in which they have been able to provide the parenting the child's requires (strengths)
- the nature of any adoptive parenting difficulties or barriers
- the changes needed to respond to the adopted child's needs more effectively and the adoptive parents view of those changes
- the support the adoptive parents need to overcome any difficulties.

Steps in analysing information about needs

Once information has been collected about the child's developmental needs, adoptive parenting capacity and relevant family and environmental factors, analysing that information forms the next stage of the assessment process. In making an analysis and assessment of the needs of the adoptive child and family, the worker should then ask a number of questions in the following sequence, taking care not to confuse needs with interventions at this stage and remembering to identify strengths as well as difficulties throughout:

1   What are the developmental needs of the child? Where is the child in terms of their development?

For example do they have health needs or problems? How is their emotional and behavioural development progressing? Are they able to manage their self-care appropriate to their age and stage of development?

2   How far are these needs arising from the adopted child's own characteristics and past history?

Sometimes the needs arise from characteristics of the adopted children themselves, for example, their genetic make-up, genetically inherited conditions, any impairments they may have. Adopted children also import a history of experiences that affect their developmental needs. What needs do they have as a result of their experiences in their birth family or subsequent placements?

3   How far do the different needs of the adopted child interrelate?

For example, an adopted child who with attachment difficulties will often have problems with poor concentration and establishing peer relationships at school, and may need support in developing family and social relationships successfully.

4   How is the adoptive parenting the child is receiving contributing to the child's needs being met or not being met?

Adoptive parents need the same core parenting skills as other parents, but they also require enhanced parenting skills to be able to respond to the extra and special needs of adopted children. Whether adopted child's needs are being met may be linked to the way their adoptive parents care for them. For example, whether adoptive parents are able to manage guidance and boundaries effectively in relation to the child's needs, or how issues of ensuring safety or providing stimulation are handled for a child with learning difficulties. The adoptive parents may have support needs of their own which relate to the task of parenting the adopted child. For example, do adoptive parents have training needs?

5 Are there any family and environmental factors that are having an impact on the care the adoptive parents can offer and/or on the needs of the adopted child?

For example, are these factors to do with the adoptive family's history that are relevant to the adopted child's needs? Is family functioning in the adoptive family affecting the child's needs or the adoptive parents' capacity to meet the needs of the child? What is the nature of the relationships with the wider adoptive family? If there is contact, with the adopted child's birth family or significant other people from their past, what is the nature of that contact and what impact does it have on the child's development needs and the adoptive parenting? Does the family have housing or financial difficulties/issues that are affecting their ability to meet the adopted child's needs? What are the strengths of the adoptive parents, their wider family and the community in which they are living?

On the basis of this analysis, the worker can gain a full understanding of the interrelated needs of the adopted child and family, and birth family members where relevant. The worker can then identify the support or interventions that would help to meet those needs and a support package for the adopted child and adoptive family, and birth relatives where appropriate, can be planned with those concerned. It is also important to identify what outcomes would indicate that the intervention has been successful.

Case example – assessing the needs of an adopted child and family and identifying appropriate support/interventions

Kate, aged 10, was the youngest of three, with older sisters Jane, aged 14, and Kelly aged 17. As a result of a series of abusive episodes, all three children had been placed six years earlier (when Kate was 4) with foster carers, who subsequently adopted them. Twice yearly contact with the birth parents had always had something of a party atmosphere, with the birth parents minimising the factors that led to the children being placed in care originally.

The adoptive parents approached the Social Services Department, who had continued to supervise contact, because of difficulties with Kate's behaviour, which were particularly marked around contact times. Her behaviour was challenging, particularly towards her adoptive father, and she rejected her adoptive mother's attempt to look after her, tended to refuse to change her clothes, hoarded objects in her room such as food, and had anxieties about being contaminated. She also appeared to be very low in mood.

Assessment

An assessment of Kate's mental health using the *Strengths and Difficulties Questionnaire* (DoH et al. 2000a) indicated that she had considerable needs, with particularly high scores on the emotional problems and pro-social scales. Her adoptive parents described the way that Kate was very caring about much younger children and animals. She often talked about her anxieties about her birth parents, especially her birth father, wanting to be sure that he would take his medication. Asked about her low mood, Kate said she felt very sad and could not care less whether she was alive or dead. She revealed she was preoccupied with thoughts about her birth parents, particularly after she had visited them, and that she and her older sister Jane had been phoning them secretly. The situation appeared to be worse since Kelly had moved away to go to college, which made Kate feel very isolated. She was confused about why she had been adopted, and why her birth parents were not able to look after her. Although an attempt had been made through the life-book to explain the reasons she was not living with her birth parents, she had few early memories, mainly focusing on the party atmosphere of their current contact. She described the fact that she was literally living with her birth parents in her mind, and seemed not to have processed the loss and to have made a new primary attachment to her adoptive parents.

Using the *Family Assessment* (Bentovim and Bingley Miller 2001) involving the two girls still at home and the adoptive parents emphasised the identity difficulties for both Kate and Jane. They felt caught between being members of the adoptive family and their birth family, Jane having more memories than Kate. The girls tended to squabble rather than support each other, creating an alliance through opposition rather than collaboration. Jane was vulnerable educationally, and had a statement. Kate was perceived as not working to her true potential and was observed to be unhappy and miserable and self-isolating in school. Although Kate presented herself well, taking care with her hair and clothes, she would insist on dressing in a grubby coat, socks unchanged and a shabby-looking top and appeared to want to present herself as poorly looked after, orphan-like. The assessment was that while she had good self-care skills, she deliberately did not use them at times to emphasis her sense of sadness, loss and feeling of being in an alien environment.

The parenting the adoptive parents were able to provide was assessed using the *HOME Inventory* (Cox and Walker 2002) and the *Family Assessment*. Although the adoptive parents had a good capacity for providing basic care and ensuring safety, Kate was rejecting of their care. The adoptive parents showed positive responsivity and encouragement of maturity but the emotional climate in the family was uncomfortable and often negative. The adoptive father was hurt by the negative attitudes of both the girls. The adoptive mother found it hard to understand Kate's behaviour and she was critical; conflict quickly emerged which was not well resolved. Although the adoptive parents did try to encourage and foster the children's achievements, there seemed to be confusion and differences between the parents about rules, about bedtimes, and how to manage the children's oppositional behaviour.

Meetings with the adoptive parents without the girls indicated the current distress and confusion showed by Kate had amplified some experiences of loss the adoptive mother had in her own childhood with the early death of her own mother. There were also concerns that the birth parents were reinforcing Kate and Jane's difficulties as they were moving towards adolescence by minimising the reasons the children were taken into care.

The adoptive parents recognised that Kate did have mental health needs and difficulties connected with her unresolved feelings about her birth parents. They were also aware that their difficulty at understanding the girls' behaviour and their way of dealing with conflict was unhelpful. The birth family were less able to acknowledge their role in undermining Kate and Jane's stability and it was felt that there would have to be far firmer boundaries around the nature of contact.

Support/intervention

Following a referral to the CAMHS Team, family therapy with the family focused on assisting the adoptive parents, first, to develop parenting approaches to deal with the challenging behaviour which both girls were showing, based on an understanding of the girls' difficulties in the context of their adoption, and second, to talk more with the girls about their early life, the reasons they came into care and their sense of sadness about their birth parents. This improved family relationships and helped to reduce Kate's mood difficulties and general sense of sadness. Careful joint work with Kate and her adoptive mother based on updating her lifestory book together proved an effective way of helping Kate process her sense of loss and unresolved feelings further and building a more positive bond between them. The adoptive mother was given the opportunity to talk through the links with her own experiences of loss. The Social Services Department took a mediating role between the adoptive parents and the birth parents to negotiate more helpful contact arrangements.

Providing support

Once the adoption order is made, the adoptive family are firmly in the driving seat and this affects the way support is provided. Some parents or young people will have clear ideas about the nature of their difficulty and the resources they would like to access. Others will have a sense that something is wrong, but be unclear about why or what might help. They will need time, a safe space and a knowledgeable social worker to talk things through and consider possible resources.

In either case, the approach of the social worker is of crucial importance. There should be a fundamental acceptance that adopters and special guardians are committed to making a unique and deeply significant contribution to the wellbeing and future development of an adopted child or children who is likely to have had a troubled history, and that they are likely to have the capacity to do so, given adequate support. The *Assessment Framework* is important as a guide to thinking comprehensively about the strengths and difficulties in the adopted child, the adoptive family and the community. Of equal importance is the capacity of the social worker to engage and communicate with the family, to listen carefully to their different perspectives and to form and test hypotheses about any concerns or difficulties alongside them.

Adoptive parents see good support as being based on a sense of partnership and reciprocity, acknowledgement and empathy, open communication, feeling listened to and believed and commitment, responsiveness and reliability (O'Neil 2003). There must also be a full acknowledgement of the family's own strengths and resources. If pre-placement services have been delivered in this spirit, it is likely that parents will be receptive to post-placement support and feel confident to seek help later on if required. Continuity of approach or worker, pre- and post-placement, is therefore important. When interventions have been considered and agreed, they should be focused, timely, positive and strengthening to individuals and to the family as a whole.

Adopted children have contact with a range of agencies in the community once they join an adoptive family, including health visitors, general practitioners, school nurses, nursery staff and teachers. These professionals have an important responsibility in identifying adopted children and families who may be in need of support services and recommending them to request an assessment for needs for support services from social services. Similarly, responding to the needs of adopted children may require services from agencies other than social services or in combination with social services help. Inter-agency work starts when an assessment of support needs is requested and involves setting up joint or parallel assessment arrangements with other professionals and agencies, as appropriate, and determining which types of intervention are most likely to be effective in responding to which needs.

In a small number of cases, post-adoption support can take on another layer of complexity. Some adopted children, even after many years in placement and a good deal of support, may remain angry and/or detached from the adoptive family. For some adoptive parents, this produces feelings of anger towards the adopted child who cannot meet their hopes and at the same time, strong feelings of guilt and inadequacy as parents. The importance of a safe and trusting relationship with the support worker cannot be over-stated in such cases and can ultimately be the single most important strand of support in sustaining the placement. Workers in such cases require skilled and regular supervision.

There remains the possibility that, even with a high level of support, an adoptive family is ultimately unable to adequately meet the needs of an adopted child on a day-to-day basis. Nevertheless, the assumption that this is a 'family for life' should underpin the approach to all adoptive family members, even in the small number of cases where adopted children eventually go to live elsewhere.

Sources of support

Informal support

Informal support networks (family, friends, community groups) will already have been identified during the preparation and Home Study period. The *Attachment Style Interview for Adoption and Fostering* is particularly helpful in identifying adopters' attachment style, their close support figures, their views about their support systems and how they use them (Bifulco et al. 2002a, 2002b). These may need to be activated or adjusted to suit the needs of the adopted child. Some parents may value help in establishing new sources of informal support through individual links with other adopters or special guardians or through agency-led groups or family days. Membership of national and regional groups can be very helpful in providing support, advice, information and local meetings.

Formal support – universal services

Adoptive parents usually obtain support for health needs through the GP, and educational issues are taken up by the adoptive parents through an approach to the school in the first instance. These universal services which promote children's mental health may be referred to as Tier 1 CAMHS. The role of the agency may be to support adoptive parents in seeking advice or to help education and health professionals to understand and respond sensitively to the adopted child's difficulties. The agency medical adviser and education adviser (if existing) can be helpful mediators. Some aspects of the school curriculum, such as genetics, sex education and family trees, can be stressful to children who are separated from their birth families. Adoptive parents may need to be forewarned regarding these issues and teachers can benefit from specific advice on dealing with them in the classroom (Adoption UK 2000).

Formal support – specialist services

Formal support through the agency should be easily accessible and continuity of social worker should be maintained wherever possible and wished for by the family. The first line of support which should be considered are the Adoption Support Services provided by the local authority. These are

- financial support
- support groups for adoptive families
- assistance with contact arrangements between adopted children and their birth relatives
- therapeutic services for adopted children
- services to ensure the continuance of adoptive relationships, including training to help meet special needs of the child and short breaks
- advice, counselling and information
- services to assist where a disruption has occurred or is in danger of occurring
- an adoption support services adviser to help those affected by adoption to access support services.

Access to specialist adoption services may be required from the outset, or later on. Adoptive parents need access to information about the sources of help open to them so that they can make informed choices they would find most helpful. Adoption agencies may feel it would be helpful to have a leaflet about the sources and types of support available. In some areas these specialist adoption services may be available within CAMHS or it may be necessary to commission services from more specialist agencies.

Within primary care, at Tier 1, the professionals who can make a contribution to the adopted child's mental health include the GP, practice and school nurses, health visitor and all the school staff including the special educational needs coordinator

(SENCO) and the local social services department. Families should be assisted in the setting up of local professional networks to support them in the care of their child and professionals need to be appraised of the adopted child's status or their needs, especially if the placement has meant a change of school and residential area. Adopted children often require the assessment or treatment of paediatricians and paramedical professionals, including occupational therapists, physiotherapists, speech and language therapists, within the context of the Child Development Team.

Tier 2 CAMHS teams have staff from a range of multidisciplinary backgrounds, including social workers, psychologists, occupational therapists and nurses. They undertake short-term work with adopted children and families. In many areas, CAMHS primary mental health workers, Tier 2 but attached to Tier 3 services, offer consultation, training and face-to-face contact work to Tier 1 services within primary care settings, including local authority looked after children's teams, general practices and schools.

Tier 3 CAMHS teams are more specialist and in some areas, there is specific provision for looked after and adopted children, usually in collaboration with Social Services, who contribute funding and/or staffing. This ensures that priority is given to these complex, time-consuming and multi-agency cases. Families particularly value being seen by professionals in teams who have expertise with adoption issues.

Model of adoption support – a specialist adoption clinic

In one Tier 3 CAMHS team all adopted children, whatever the presenting problem, are seen in the specialist Adoption Clinic. All staff working in the clinic receive training on adoption and attachment issues and specialist supervision. An adoption-friendly model of assessment is used including routinely seeing adoptive parents without their adopted children during the assessment, being aware of and openly acknowledging the differences that adoption brings to the family, and the significance of pre-placement history of the adopted child. An effort is made to understand what difficulties the child brought with them into the family and how these are influencing the presenting problems. Interventions will often involve supporting adoptive parents with appropriate parenting strategies for adopted children with attachment difficulties, focusing on facilitating attachment relationship by including the adoptive parents in therapy sessions with the child, and liaising with schools to help their understanding of adopted children with identity and relationship difficulties.

Tier 4 CAMHS teams are available for the small number of adopted children and young people who have such severe difficulties that they may require inpatient assessment and treatment or specialist day services for a period of time. They may also require specialist therapeutic or educational services provided outside local authority provision. Decisions of this kind would need to be made in the context of a multi-agency care plan following an initial referral to Tier 3 services.

Case example – specialist assessment and therapy

Assessment

A Social Services Department (SSD) had placed Bethany and Gary with adoptive parents eighteen months previously, when they were 4 and 2 years old respectively. The children had had very disturbing experiences living with their mentally ill birth mother. Although the adoptive parents, James and Amanda, were completely committed to both children they realised very early on that they were both extremely emotionally disturbed and this was reflected in their very challenging behaviour, which was exhausting to live with. The placing social worker offered what support she could but soon felt out of her depth. James and Amanda did not feel they should proceed with the adoption until they had been provided with a specialist assessment and therapy. They had attended seminars and read widely and knew there were independent specialist assessment services for adoptive families such as theirs. Social services agreed to fund such an assessment which highlighted that both children had significant attachment difficulties.

Support/intervention

There was a recommendation for an intensive five-day programme involving the whole family. The SSD agreed funding. The family had the support of a therapy team of four specially trained therapists throughout the five days. The focus of the work was on helping the family develop a more coherent narrative about the children's past and to begin to facilitate healthier attachment relationships. There was plenty of opportunity to give time to the parents and children separately as well as together. Amanda and James were able to increase their understanding of how the children's attachment disturbance was affecting their parenting and to learn different strategies for managing them. Some of the family work involved creative therapies to graphically dramatise the effects of certain traumatic incidents in the children's lives. It was a powerful emotional experience and one that was a turning point. Amanda and James know there is no miracle cure for their children but the therapy they experienced gave them confidence and much greater understanding of the special parenting Bethany and Gary needed from them. The promise of a two-year follow-up programme from the same team of therapist helped them make the commitment to proceed with the adoption (Archer and Burnell 2003).

A coordinated approach to support

In some cases, adopted children may require a wide range of services from different agencies. These could include child mental health services, child development or paediatric services, social work support (including for contact arrangements), short breaks, baby/child sitting and special education provision. It is important that such services are provided in an integrated, child-centred way.

Case example – inter-agency working

Jamie, a 6-year-old adopted child with a number of disabilities, had a wide range of professionals involved with his care. A child's worker held an annual meeting of the adoptive parents and all the professionals involved with an adopted child with disabilities and his family. This allowed for an exchange of information between Jamie's adoptive parents, as experts on the child's care, and the various professionals who provided different aspects of the child's care. The meeting formed a basis for ironing out any difficulties and planning ahead for the next year (Argent 2003a).

Liaison between agencies at a strategic level is required to facilitate a coordinated approach to service delivery at the level of individual adopted children and families. Workers should aim to create a package of care that meets all of the adopted child's needs and should be able to identify the appropriate referral routes in their area in order to achieve this.

Local authorities vary in the way in which they provide services for children and adults with disabilities. Whatever the arrangements, adoptive parents should be given clear information about procedures and practices of various departments and they should know whom to contact for each element of their services (DfES 2005a).

A coordinated, inter-agency approach is essential to meet adopted children's needs and is embedded in current government policy (Rushton 2003a, 2003b; Rushton and Dance 2003). With the implementation of *Every Child Matters* (DfES 2003a) and the Children Act 2004, when children are in contact with more than one professional at a time, there should be a single professional coordinating their services, providing continuity and building trust. For adopted children, the ASSA may have a role in identifying an appropriate worker or even acting as that lead professional.

Model of adoption support – Inter-agency Adoption Support Forum

In one city an Inter-agency Adoption Support Forum with representatives from Child Health, Child and Adolescent Mental Health, Social Services, Education, and local voluntary organisations involved in adoption work meet together three times a year for both information sharing and planning training and developments. The forum has contributed through discussion and support to the development of a short breaks care scheme specifically designed for adoptive families and a supported lodgings scheme for adopted young people set up be agencies represented in the forum. Teamwork and an interagency approach are essential in working with individual families, which needs to be supported by joined up thinking at the strategic planning level. Both these schemes grew out of the needs and demands from adoptive families for these services.

FORMS OF SUPPORT

There is a range of areas within which support services are likely to be required. These can be grouped under the following headings:

- providing information, practical support and financial support
- the development of an adoptive identity
- parenting adopted children with behavioural and emotional difficulties
- contact with birth families.

Each of these areas will be considered in terms of the types of support and interventions that might be offered.

Providing information, practical support and financial support

The provision of financial and other practical support to adopters and special guardians is extremely important although professionals have often regarded it as a lower priority (Rushton and Dance 2003).

Providing information

The provision of accurate information to adoptive parents and special guardians is of vital importance at all levels. Full and detailed information about the adopted child and the child's background should be shared at all stages of the matching process and adoptive parents may wish to have access to it at different stages later on. New information about birth family members should be passed on wherever possible.

Adoptive parents should have access to full medical information and, where necessary, advice from health professionals about their adopted child's health needs, medical treatment and likely future health needs. Some parents may continue to need support when there is uncertainty about future physical and mental health needs, or issues may arise unexpectedly, later on.

There are a wide range of publications and resources that are relevant to both adoptive parents and children. Particularly helpful for adoptive parents are books that focus on general adoption issues (Morris 1999; Salter 2002; Van Gulden and Bartels-Rabb 1995), parenting troubled children (Archer 2000a, 2000b; Cairns 2002; Jewett 1995) and talking about adoption (Chennells and Morrison 1998). For adopted children, stories connected with adoption (Byrne and Chambers 1997a, 1997b, 1999; Foxon 2001), and books and resources that cover 'life story' areas (Betts and Ahmad 2003; Camis 2001) can be helpful as different issues arise through their growing up. Adoptive parents also need to be kept informed of local training workshops, groups and social events which they can attend.

Training is a key part of an adoption support service (Argent 2003b). Adoptive parents may wish to be offered training either at the point of placement or in the future. It is important to find out whether the new parents wish to be included in the adoption agency's training programme or to be funded for other programmes relating to their adopted child's special needs. New adoptive parents cannot predict all their training needs but the right to training should be agreed.

Practical support

There are many forms of practical support that may be helpful to adopters, special guardians and their children at different times throughout the family life cycle.

Practical assistance with specific tasks can be particularly welcome at times. For instance, help with administrative tasks such as completing forms, making telephone calls or writing letters may be beneficial. Some families may need the help of an interpreter.

When adopted children have physical or learning disabilities, workers should ensure that they have all the aids and adaptations to which they are entitled, including incontinence services (Argent 2003a).

Caring for disabled children can be physically and emotionally exhausting and adoptive parents will need to take occasional breaks. This can also be the case for adopted children with more severe emotional and behavioural difficulties. Friends and family care may not be available or suitable sources of help and child sitting and short break schemes can be invaluable in allowing adoptive parents to know that their children are safely and appropriately cared for. Such schemes should be included as part of the support agenda, whether or not adoptive parents feel them to be necessary, as this makes it easier for people to change their minds later on. It is important that schemes are tailored to individual needs as far as possible (Argent 2003b).

Case example – finding the right support

Assessment

To begin with, Jane and Michael didn't want to leave Rosie with anyone else, but when they felt more confident about controlling her fits, no one they knew was willing to take responsibility for a whole evening. They didn't want to go back to the agency because nothing had been said about babysitting. They were worried about being seen as failures, because they had told the social worker that they had a supportive network of family and friends. So they just stopped going out together until a researcher picked up what was happening.

Support/intervention

The researcher helped them to make a successful application to social services for a medically trained babysitter (Argent and Kerrane 1997).

Financial support

In the process of working through the dimensions in Chapters 5, 6 and 7, and in particular the section on Income in Chapter 7, the worker may have identified a number of new forms of expenditure that will be incurred by the adoptive family in relation to the adoptive child who lives with them. In most situations we expect that an actual service is the best way of meeting an identified need, but it is also the case that financial payments may be necessary to cover the costs of maintaining an adoptive child, purchasing specific goods and also on occasion paying for a service.

There are two key issues to consider before these financial needs can be translated into a recommendation by the assessor for a financial payment to be made. First, Regulation 8 of the 2005 Regulations states the circumstances under which financial support can be paid. These are set out above.

Second, for certain specified forms of expenditure as listed in Regulation 15(6) of the Adoption Support Services Regulations 2005, the means of the adoptive family do not need to be (and in some cases must not be) taken into account before payment amounts are made. But for most payments the local authority is required, when deciding on the amount it will pay, to have regard to the projected financial circumstances of the adoptive family and child. In effect, a means test is carried out.

In particular, any regular payments for the purposes of supporting the upkeep of the child and/or special needs expenditure need to be means tested in line with the legislative requirements. The results of this means test should then be applied to the relevant rates that their authority uses as the maximum possible payment levels to adopters (these may well be linked to the local fostering 'boarding-out' rates and enhancement payments). Each local authority will have its own guides on carrying out these means tests based on the Adoption Support Services Regulations and statutory guidance.

Methods of payment

Payments can be made on a regular basis and/or as a lump sum. The most frequent form of payment is an ongoing one to help an adoptive family cover the basic upkeep costs associated with the adoptive child that has joined them. Other forms of financial support are one-off or a short series of payments to contribute towards the cost of specific items which could otherwise not be afforded. Occasionally bigger homes and cars will be needed if a new child is to join a family, and financial help may be needed to facilitate this.

Adoption payments cannot include any element of remuneration, apart for foster carers who adopt in specific circumstances. As discussed in Chapter 7, payments can also not duplicate any tax credit or benefit that the adoptive family is entitled to.

Model of adoption support – a welfare benefits adviser as adoption support

Some agencies have access to a welfare benefits adviser whom adoptive parents and staff can consult about the statutory rights about leave and pay, benefits and grants benefits and other financial support issues.

The development of an adoptive identity

Children who are adopted or cared for by special guardians need to form a positive sense of their identity, based on realistic understandings of their life stories and the acknowledgement of two sets of parents. This is a lifelong task and the significance and meaning of an adoptive identity will change and vary in intensity over time.

Adoption services should be alert to the importance of identity building at all stages of the adoption process. It is essential that full and detailed background information be gathered on behalf of all adopted children. This will enable them to be introduced to the facts of their adoption and gradually helped to understand their birth family and cultural heritage.

Background information needs to be balanced and accurate, neither glossing 'difficult' information nor neglecting to include positive information (Ryan and Walker 1999). The widespread practice of putting together lifestory books and collecting personal memorabilia for adopted children helps with this task. ASSAs have an important role in advising other workers about the preparation of lifestory books. It is important to bear in mind the developmental stage of the adopted child and to avoid information that is too complex for them to absorb. Young adopted children can benefit from a book of photographs with simple captions, with more complicated and potentially painful information being held separately for later use.

Adoptive parents may feel less excluded as parents if they can actively help to research the adopted child's history and/or be supported to keep the lifestory book up-to-date and age appropriate (Sykes 2000). This of course needs to be at a pace and a level which helps to give the child greater understanding without disrupting the process of becoming identified with the adoptive family and their cultural context. It is important to remember that the birth family history will continue to evolve after placement and new information about births, deaths, health and other significant changes may need to be incorporated into the adopted child's story.

Adopted children may need to develop a 'story' that conveys the information they wish to give and with which they feel comfortable. Adoptive parents may need advice on helping a child to construct a narrative, or different narratives to use in different social situations. Sometimes, children (including birth children) in an adoptive family may need to be helped to prepare responses to queries about the nature and composition of their family.

If the adopted child's background story is particularly unusual or painful, adopters and special guardians may need support and advice from the agency on how best to disclose the information to them. Young people may also need personal support or therapeutic help at this time.

Model of adoption support – gathering information

An adoption support project in a voluntary agency offers a service where 'child appreciation days' are organised and led at the point of matching for the adopted child. The purpose is to bring the child and their history to life for the prospective adopters in a way that descriptions written in adult language on forms may not. Invitations are sent to professionals and any significant adults including carers from the child's past including birth family members where appropriate. Those attending bring memorabilia and photographs for retention by the child and the adoptive parents, and the leader takes participants on a conducted journey where a child-centred account of the child's life is recounted by the participants, with particular emphasis on filling gaps. Family trees and flow charts of significant events and moves can be completed and the day is written up as a story from the perspective of the child. These days also promote the development of informal networks between people significant to the adopted child.

When adopters can create an open atmosphere and can talk about the birth family in a balanced way, this is likely to lead to better outcomes for the adopted child. This is important not only for adopted children who are in contact with birth relatives, but also (and possibly even more so) for children who cannot, for whatever reason, retain links with birth relatives (Jaffee and Fanshel 1970; McWhinnie 1967; Raynor 1980; Triseliotis 1973).

Support offered to adoptive parents should be focused on building their capacity to empathise with the identity needs of their adopted child that arise because they are adopted and with the child's birth family. If adoptive parents are not able to feel some empathy with the birth family they are unlikely to be able to help an adopted child develop a positive sense of their identity. This includes their identity as a member of their adoptive family, integrating their important heritage with a birth family and yet being realistic about what has happened to them (Neil 2002).

Support interventions which may be helpful for adoptive parents in helping them talk about difficult issues with their adopted child include the following (Neil 2003):

- helping the adoptive parents find the words to tell the child their story
- making sure they have enough information abut the child's history which has not only facts but also a qualitative sense of the circumstances and lives of the birth family at the time
- helping them make sense of that information themselves by giving them frameworks for explaining the birth parents' behaviour in relation to, for example, the impact of abuse, substance misuse, mental health difficulties and the birth parents' own history
- helping them to understand their child's need to be able to express mixed feelings about birth family members.

Sometimes it is helpful to take a family approach to providing support when an adopted child is struggling to assimilate difficult information from the past into their adoptive identity. Lifestory books may be reviewed, created or built on during family sessions. This approach can help adopted children to order their experiences, link past and present and express their fantasies, hopes and expectations alongside their adoptive parents. Pictorial timelines, where adopted children are helped to represent, through drawings or paintings, the significant people in their lives, may also be helpfully created in family sessions. The *In My Shoes* (Calam et al. 2000) interview can be used to review with the child, and adoptive parents where helpful, their feelings and views about aspects of their history and their current life. Therapeutic rituals which have meaning for all family members, such as candle lighting rituals, planting trees and so on can help celebrate and strengthen adoptive family ties as well as validating connections to a birth family and help an adopted child cope with loss. Journal writing and role-playing can be useful for teenagers, who may be encouraged to write a letter to a birth parent sharing wishes and feelings and then take the role of a birth parent and draft a response (Brodzinsky et al. 1998).

Some adopted children need individual counselling or therapy as they become more aware of the losses that are inherent in adoption. Issues that were accepted without question in early childhood can give rise to anxiety as children's thinking processes and general awareness increase. They may need help to express a sense of loss, rejection or abandonment, to be reassured of the permanence of adoption or to fill in some of the detail and gain a more mature understanding of why they were separated from their biological families.

Model of adoption support – a resource pack for adopters to help with telling children about their family and heritage

A 'resource pack' can be compiled by agencies to help adopters' capacities to talk openly and easily about sensitive and complex information, about their own histories and the adopted child's history. This contains ideas, research findings and practice guidance, to be used by both workers and adoptive parents and might include the following:

* Making age-appropriate books, magazine and newspaper articles available to the adopted person.
* Story-telling – use fictional characters to relate the experiences of the adopted child to stimulate dialogue and discussion.
* Playing – use of art materials, dolls or role-play to give children an appropriate medium in which to explore and express their thoughts and feelings.
* Acknowledging that it is natural to have questions and let children know that you are willing to answer all you can.
* Making appropriately positive comments about the birth family so that the adopted child has a sense that the birth family (but not what they did, if maltreatment is part of the history) is accepted by the adoptive family.
* Laying down knowledge and the whereabouts of significant people who might be to be contacted as sources of information about the adopted child's early life.
* Providing information leaflets containing advice about the talking and telling process.
* Sensitising teachers, doctors and other family and health core professionals to adoption issues helping them to regard as normal adopted people's interest and questions about their birth family.
* Making visits to the adopted child's area of origin (Feast and Howe 2003).

It may be easy to believe that an adopted child with severe learning difficulties cannot comprehend their own story but opportunities for telling it should never be overlooked. Sometimes an imaginative approach is needed to help a child understand their background in a way that they can understand and respond to. Helping adoptive parents communicate with their disabled child has to be part of adoption support and adoption support has to be part of a learning loop whereby workers can learn from adoptive parents what works and what does not work and how to improve the service they offer.

Case example – lifestory work with a disabled adopted child

Assessment

Andy, aged 11, had seen his mother taken away in an ambulance when he was 4. He had very serious learning difficulties and general developmental delay. He was placed with kind foster carers. He wasn't told when his mother died and he wasn't taken to the funeral. He certainly would not have had any concept about death. He probably thought that she had left him because he made her cross – she had sometimes left him alone in the flat when she was upset. Andy made little progress while in the foster home. After a year, Andy was placed with a single prospective adopter. She thought it was important for Andy to be told his story even if he did not understand it.

Support/intervention

She talked about his mother and wrote a simple narrative about his life, which she illustrated with photographs and read to him every night. Finally, she took him to see his mother's grave. Only then did he stop waiting for his mother to come back and look after him. From that time on, he could begin to make progress in his new family (Argent 2003a).

For children and families from ethnic minorities, support regarding identity issues should include a thorough understanding of racism and its impact on the psychological wellbeing of all black children as well as the particular issues of adoption and fostering. Services for black and minority ethnic children should form part of a wider overall agency approach which includes consideration of issues for staffing, language, resources and skills, community links and a full commitment to inclusion throughout the agency (Charlton et al. 1998; Harris 2005; Sellick et al. 2004).

Therapeutic approaches designed to help adopted children and families with identity issues should be adapted to the specific needs and experience of black and minority ethnic adopted children and families. This includes not only involving people from the wider family and social networks who are significant to the adopted child, when appropriate, but also ensuring that empowerment (important for all adopted children) is a key focus in the approaches used in work with families (Duck 2003).

For transracially adopted young people, services may be provided proactively given the difficulties that it is known that this group can experience (Harris 2003). Group work and individual counselling through specialist organisations may be helpful (Dance and Rushton 2005a). It may also be important to identify people, activities or groups or schools in the area who could assist in helping these young people to develop a positive sense of their cultural identity.

Model of adoption support – a service for black, adopted young people

A voluntary agency has developed services to address the specific needs and concerns of black, adopted young people. The service emphasises the value of mutual support in allowing this group of adopted young people who face similar potentially isolating and specific challenges to talk and share activities together. It runs groups and workshops to facilitate this. Young people have valued these opportunities to talk through the difficulties they have encountered in establishing their sense of self, both as adopted children in the face of racism and ambivalence about adoption (Chamberlain and Horne 2003).

Parenting adopted children with behavioural and emotional problems

Adoptive parents and special guardians can find themselves seriously challenged by their adopted child's behaviour and emotional distress. It is important to develop working partnerships with adoptive parents and adopted children that take full account of the impact of the adopted child's history and/or their genetic inheritance and the pressures that the ensuing difficulties can place on family life. When difficulties become more extreme, adoptive parents may become isolated and lose confidence in themselves. It is important that they feel accepted and empowered as 'good enough parents' and that they regain the belief that they have a key role in helping their adopted child to recover (Gordon 2003).

Settling in and creating a new family

The early weeks of placement can be an extremely vulnerable time for adopted children and their new families, with many practical and psychological adjustments to be made (Dance and Rushton 2005a; Rushton and Dance 2004). It is important to offer regular, frequent and sensitive support, ideally from a familiar social worker who knows the family well. Transitions can be eased by

- good information sharing prior to placement
- working in partnership with foster carers to ensure that they are supportive of the move and can give the adopted child psychological permission to move on
- ensuring that the loss of the foster family for the adopted child is acknowledged and that bonds are not severed abruptly

- allowing all parties time to think through the move and the placement
- ensuring that all parties have, to some degree, tested out the reality of the move and feel committed to it, albeit with some ambivalence (Lowe et al. 1999), a commitment to the move.

The move to a new school is of great importance and the responsibility for organising this is commonly left with the new adoptive parents. Where there are known or potential educational issues or where new parents are inexperienced, agencies should be proactive in taking a liaison role and ensuring that the most suitable school is chosen, that the timing of the adopted child's entry is appropriate and that the child is prepared to cope with the new school experience. They can also ensure that background information is shared sensitively and that the adopted child's teacher and the school as a whole are attuned to adoption-related issues (Scott and Lindsey 2003).

In the early stages of the placement, new adoptive parents can be helped to ease the adopted child's adjustment in the following ways:

- Keeping as much continuity from the previous environment as possible, in the short term; for example, basic routines, foods, clothing etc. For babies and toddlers, the sense of smell is important and continuity can be offered in bedding, washing powder etc.
- Trying to avoid unnecessary travel and excessive numbers of visitors to the home.
- Avoiding alternative carers and sitters, and unnecessary separations from the adopted child.
- Providing additional opportunities for nurture, one-to-one caregiving, shared activities, play and gentle stimulation.
- Providing close contact, if the child is comfortable with this, or finding alternative opportunities for touch if not (swimming, games, watching television together etc).
- Setting aside a time in each day when the parent is fully focused on the adopted child and providing a shared, enjoyable experience (Archer 2000a, 2000b; Fahlberg 1994).

Support to adoptive parents

Adoptive parents often need support in understanding their adopted children's behaviours and in knowing how to respond in ways that promote their adopted child's capacity to build trusting relationships. Adoptive caregiving is usually optimal or 'adequately' sensitive and yet, in an important minority of cases, adopted children still fail to make a selective attachment. These children may need particularly finely attuned and sensitive caregiving. Adoptive parents may need intensive and compassionate support to acknowledge and cope with their own feelings of loss and disappointment while yet having to carry on with their adoptive parenting task without any obvious 'rewards'.

A detailed analysis of caregiving by long-term foster carers (Beek and Schofield 2004b; Schofield et al. 2000) provides a model of sensitive caregiving based in attachment theory (Ainsworth et al. 1978). Using this framework, sensitive care-giving can be understood as

- providing availability
- promoting reflective capacity
- building self-esteem
- promoting autonomy
- promoting family membership.

Foster carers who had skills across these dimensions of parenting were able to establish rewarding relationships with their fostered children, even when progress was very slow. These aspects of sensitive caregiving have also been identified as promoting security and good progress in children with severe learning disabilities (Beek and Schofield 2004a).

Building resilience

Resilience is enhanced when children feel connected to key people, in particular their caregivers. Resilience can also be promoted by school experiences that maximise the child's potential and by positive involvement in leisure activities, team and individual pursuits, volunteering, caring for animals, groups and so on. Adoptive parents, special guardians, social workers and other professionals engaged with the adopted child can work together to promote resilience.

Promoting peer relationships is central to the self-esteem of an adopted child and adoptive parents have a key role in strengthening children's positive attributes and relationships (Scott and Lindsey 2003). Support for adoptive parents can mean encouraging them to provide additional help to their adopted children in the area of peer relationships. This may be through bringing friends home or encouraging them to join clubs or take up activities, so that they build up a network of friends. This may involve careful supervision and guidance of time spent with peers or negotiation with local leisure and activity groups so that an adopted child's additional needs can be taken into account.

Belonging to groups for children who have similar differences, such as groups for adopted children, can help children to feel comfortable with themselves, to raise self-esteem and improve social presentation. Common issues can be shared and ways of coping can be shared. Some agencies run groups or away days for adopted children of different ages, or from ethnic minorities or with disabilities which can help them to feel a sense of belonging in a group of children with whom they have much in common.

Model of adoption support – a youth worker for young adopted people

One adoption service appointed a youth worker to work with individuals and groups. It was felt that a person from this discipline would have a good under-standing of ensuring equality of opportunity and have the ability to communicate and relate to young people. An activity day, a monthly youth club session, individual counselling and a summer activity camp were offered and all proved successful and popular. All were felt to have achieved their overall aim which was 'to provide appropriate, safe environments where adopted children and young people can feel able to explore their thoughts, feelings and experiences of adoption with each other and with workers' (Eccles 2003: 119).

Case example – promoting resilience through sport

Assessment

Anne, aged 9½, was worried about her image in school as clumsy and slow.

Support/intervention

Her sympathetic foster carers were searching for ways to try to improve her coordination and self-confidence and hit upon the idea of skiing lessons on the local dry ski slope. This turned out to be an inspired move. She proved to be a natural on the slopes and a star of her class, with an obvious knock-on effect on her self-esteem and self-belief.

Parenting work

There is a fair amount of evidence that parenting programmes used in the general population can help adoptive parents to reduce certain problematic behaviours, and this in itself can reduce stress (Scott et al. 2001). There are a variety of such programmes available and adopters and special guardians may find them helpful, particularly if they have not parented before. However, they are not 'adoption sensitive' and there will be shortfalls for adopters and special guardians.

The particular stresses of parenting children with the emotional and behavioural difficulties associated with maltreatment, separation and loss can be addressed only through more specialised approaches to enhancing adoptive parenting skills.

There are specific programmes or interventions for adoptive parents, which focus on building more positive relationships within the family. Suggested key ingredients for success of such programmes are that they are fairly lengthy (at least twenty hours of input) and that there is an emphasis on learning new practical skills (Pallett et al. 2002).

One multidisciplinary and multi-intervention programme works with the adoptive parents to make sense of troubled behaviours and to develop effective re-parenting strategies (Archer and Gordon 2004; Gordon 2003). A helpful strand of the programme, and one which can be developed as a local intervention strategy, is the use of a parent mentor (preferably an adoptive parent with the appropriate training) to assist adoptive parents in learning the 'language of trauma' reflected in a troubled child's behaviour, using a series of parenting strategies and modelling alternatives ways of communicating. This helps the child learn to lay down new neuro-biological pathways and learn new behaviours and ways of relating – i.e. the 'language of love'. There is a strong emphasis on the need for adopters to receive support, empathy and validation and encouragement for them to take care of themselves and their own needs. The programme has been evaluated as successful in helping adoptive parents to hold on to their adopted children and parent them more effectively, even if change in the children is small or very slow.

There is some evidence that the use of Webster-Stratton-based training programmes adapted for newly approved adoptive parents helps their confidence and provides them with useful parenting techniques and strategies (Gilkes and Klimes 2003). Another specific parenting course, delivered by trained adopters, uses an attachment theory framework (Adoption UK 2000). It offers support, information, parenting strategies and anger management techniques and is reported to be helpful for adopters, though it has not been independently evaluated.

Model of adoption support – multidisciplinary support for long-term carers and looked after children

A multidisciplinary project involves social workers, education and clinical psychologist working together to support long term carers and looked after children. Direct consultation sessions are provided for the carer to plan and provide support and interventions are aimed at enabling the carer to create a positive emotional atmosphere, to avoid confrontation and to set clear boundaries in an empathetic manner. Group sessions allow carers to reflect on difficulties, gain support and gain further skills and direct work with children, alongside their carers, is offered where the other approaches are not working. Evaluation of the programme indicate that carers feel more supported and especially value psychological advice and support (Golding 2003).

An intervention (based in the Netherlands), which aimed to help new adoptive parents respond more sensitively to their babies, showed proof of effectiveness (Juffer et al. 1997; Stams et al. 2001). Mother–child interactions were videoed, then played back and mothers given feedback on how they might respond more sensitively to their babies. A seven-year follow-up showed enduring effects of this intervention in terms of the emotional development of the adopted children. Such interventions are becoming increasingly trialled and used in the United Kingdom in the general population and may be a useful resource for adoptive parents with adopted babies.

Another adoption-specific programme involves the analysis of live communication between adoptive parents and adopted children. Adoptive parents are observed interacting with their adopted children and guided toward more positive approaches through a headphone. The live coaching lasts for about ten minutes, followed by a longer period of discussion. Themes of play, praise, setting limits and discipline strategies are explored (Scott and Lindsey 2003).

Some treatment approaches include the use of 'holding' techniques which involve close physical contact between the therapist or adoptive parent and adopted child, with touch and eye contact being encouraged. The approach usually involves the child being 'held', forcibly if they struggle, until they become quiet and ready to make eye contact and other communication with the person 'holding' them. These techniques were developed partly in response to an identified need to provide a more intensive form of treatment for certain adopted children with severe attachment difficulties and they aim to enable the child to develop and promote attachment behaviours, to which the caregivers can respond. One small-scale evaluation of an attachment-based intervention which included holding therapy indicated that the twelve families who received it showed a drop in problem behaviour scores compared to the eleven who received no intervention (Myeroff et al. 1999). There remains, however, very limited empirical support for these approaches (Rushton 2004).

Promoting attachments between adopted children who have attachment difficulties resulting from maltreatment and trauma a slow, long-term and very challenging process and adoptive parents need both skills, psychological understanding of the child's needs, time and a great deal of patience. If the child's difficulties are too severe, the child and family usually need a multifaceted approach with a range of different intervention approaches.

'Holding' is a form of restraint (although it is intended to be therapeutic), and has attracted considerable concern which centres on the risk of the adopted child experiencing 'holding' as intrusive, insensitive and therefore non-therapeutic, and the possibility of retraumatising the child. It is contra-indicated when a child has been physically or sexually abused. Quinton and Selwyn (2006) make the point that in empirical studies any positive outcomes may have other explanations than the treatment being investigated and they also emphasise concerns about injuries being caused. BAAF have issued a position statement on attachment disorder in which they clearly state that in their view 'agencies should not use or commission interventions generally termed holding therapy' and argue that there are serious issues with withdrawing consent (2006). Given the lack of evidence and the concerns surrounding this form on intervention, 'holding' should not be undertaken without considerable caution as a treatment for children who have attachment difficulties. If such treatments are being considered, it will, of course, be essential to obtain the informed consent of the adopted child or young person concerned and their adoptive parents, and for those undertaking the treatment to have appropriate training and supervision so that safety issues have been taken into account.

Adoptive parents are often anxious to find forms of treatment which might help them and their adopted children, some of which lie outside conventional therapeutic approaches. We, like BAAF, would have serious concerns about supporting any treatment approaches with an uncertain evidential base and about which there was serious professional disagreement. As with all forms of therapy, it is important that adoptive parents have access to adequate information about the risks and benefits involved. ASSAs may wish to consult with colleagues in CAMHS teams for advice.

Behavioural treatments

Specific behavioural treatments can be effective, especially if they are part of a wider package of support to the family (Scott and Lindsey 2003). Particular behaviours (for example, bed wetting and soiling, specific fears and phobias) are focused upon and caregivers encouraged to record them, along with the precursors and events that follow. Different responses are then proposed and tested. Progress in such defined areas can help adoptive parents to feel more effective and adopted children to feel more successful, and can result in a general improvements in relationships.

There is also evidence that cognitive behavioural and dynamic approaches can help to ameliorate the effects of trauma. The approach helps to develop coping strategies to deal with emotional responses. These are achieved by talking through of negative events and developing understanding and alternative ways of explaining what happened (Bentovim 2004). This process may be necessary prior to place-ment so that adopted children can allow themselves to have more satisfying relationships in their new families

Family therapy

The focus of intervention in family therapy is the relationships between family members, rather than individual difficulties. When applied to adoptive families, it is important that adoptive parents do not feel themselves 'blamed' for the difficul-ties they are experiencing. The adopted child should be viewed in the context of earlier harmful life experiences and it should be acknowledged that family relations have been put under stress by the troubled behaviours that the adopted child has brought into the family. Explorations of the origins of the child's difficulties can be helpful. Family therapy can be productive in addressing the day-to-day issues of family relations, especially when accompanied by more specific advice on behav-iour management. It can also provide a safe setting in which adopted children can be helped to explore their earlier experiences in the presence of their new adoptive parents (Scott and Lindsey 2003).

Peer support

Adoptive parents can feel deskilled and rejected when adopted children do not allow them to get close or when troubled behaviours persist over time. This may create confusion and frustration, which is hard to express to non-adoptive parents. These feelings are important targets for intervention in their own right and support groups are helpful in this respect. Peer support can be invaluable in helping adoptive parents to realise that they are not alone and that their experiences are 'normal' in the broad context of adoption (Chamberlain and Horne 2003). Individual links with adoptive parents in similar situations can also be productive.

Gaining support from other adoptive parents via national and international Internet communication has been found to be helpful (O'Connor and Zeanah 2003; Rushton and Dance 2003). In inter-country adoption the Internet offers the possi-bility of being in contact with a worldwide peer group of adopted children and adoptive parents.

Model of adoption support – using a website for providing adoption support

One adoption agency created a website to link up social services staff, foster carers and adoptive parents and looked after and adopted children. This enabled the provision of e-support, the establishment of an e-community and communication in a large rural community and alternatives to traditional educational and training opportunities (Sellick and Howell 2003).

Personal support

Adopted children with emotional and behavioural difficulties can sometimes have the effect of reactivating past emotional issues in their caregivers. For instance, a grieving adopted child can reawaken the pain of unresolved loss in the parent's past. Adopters and special guardians may sometimes need individual specialist help in order to be able to offer their child emotional responsiveness. It is the responsibility of an adoption support service to be able to identify sources of counselling or therapy for adoptive parents if it is felt to be necessary.

Support for adopted children

Individual therapy

Studies which have followed placements for several years after adopted child joined new family suggest that therapeutic intervention directly with the child in the first second year of placement may not always be appropriate (Sellick et al. 2004). However, many adopted children gain great benefit from sustaining a relationship with a therapist who has been previously involved and has seen them through the transition to a new placement. Adopted children's needs for therapy must be assessed individually and in partnership with their adoptive parents or special guardians.

Adopted children of all ages can benefit from a safe space in which to talk or play and, in doing so, explore their intense and often contradictory feelings about people and events from the past. Therapeutic work should always occur in the context of ongoing work with the adoptive parents and with attention to other aspects of the adopted child's life especially school (Scott and Lindsey 2003).

Adopted children can be helped to process and let go of frightening or painful memories and associations through individual play therapy, psychotherapy or group therapy. Work with children in transition from foster care to adoption can be especially relevant and helpful when they are facing the enormous stress of losing trusted caregivers while simultaneously being expected to form new relationships (Lanyando 2003).

Case example – individual therapy

Assessment

Sammy, a 7-year-old adopted child, was tormented by his memories of life with his birth parents. He had been a carer for them and his younger sister and worried about their safety now. He had vivid flashbacks of abusive experiences and he so feared the return of the abuser that he kept his curtains drawn.

Support/intervention

In his treatment, Sammy gradually found a way to articulate the many contradictory emotions that were inhibiting his capacity for friendship and adversely affecting his function in school.

Recognising and naming feelings

Children with a history of abuse and neglect can be re-alerted to sensations of touch, taste, smell and sight through therapeutic games and exercises. They can be helped to recognise and name feelings of hunger, pain and tiredness as well as emotions such as happy, sad and angry. When these sensations can be accurately named and understood, they are less likely to trigger inappropriate behaviours. A growing awareness of feelings and associated memories allows children to make more sense of difficult relationship experiences and to handle current relationship in a more balanced and constructive way. There are a range of tools for helping children identify and name their feelings and to learn to communicate what they feel when with different people and in different situations. *In My Shoes* (Calam et al. 2000) is an effective tool for this work with children and their adoptive parents.

Cognitive behavioural therapy

A cognitive behavioural approach can be effective in helping adolescent children to manage their anger more effectively. Anger can erupt if children anticipate a hostile reaction from others. They can learn to identify the triggers and circumstances that generate anger and to plan responses that are less conflictual. They can also learn relaxation techniques to use at these times.

Model of adoption support – using play therapy techniques

An innovative use of play therapy techniques pioneered by one adoption support agency has proved effective in addressing adoptive parents' concerns about the adopted child's behavioural difficulties, and at the same time, significantly improving the relationship and attachment between the parent and the child. Two experienced play therapists provide a six-month programme that begins with a parent receiving weekly training in play therapy techniques at workshops that do not include the child. Subsequently, the parent provides 'special play times' at a regular time and place with the child, receiving regular support and feedback about the sessions from the play therapist. Significantly, the most usual impact is that the parent develops greater understanding of the meaning and significance of the behaviour for the child and is thus more able to tolerate and manage it. This change can diminish threat of exclusion from the adoptive family, as, in tandem with the reduction in distress and tension, the behaviour can change for the better. In addition to professional supervision of the play sessions and access to telephone consultation, support groups for adoptive parents working in this way are provided (Howe et al. 1999).

Contact with birth families

Maintaining indirect and face-to-face contact arrangements is a complex task that adoptive and birth families may need support to manage. It should be assumed that adoptive and birth families might need regular discussions with ASSAs or others about their feelings and responses to the contact as these will change over time. Voluntary contract agreements agreed by all parties can provide a useful basis for planning and reviewing contact arrangements.

Contact arrangements may need to be renegotiated because of the changing developmental needs of the adopted child or changing adoptive or birth family circumstances. Support services should be responsive to such requests. If appropriate, a family meditation model can be helpful in negotiating a new agreement.

Indirect contact

Indirect contact is increasingly built into plans for adopted children and in many cases it is a successful means of keeping the door open between the adoptive family and the birth family. An efficient, highly confidential, user-friendly and well-monitored 'post box' service is necessary to facilitate satisfactory indirect contact.

However, indirect contact may require further support post-placement as a range of difficulties can occur. Written communication can provide opportunities for people to misinterpret each other (Grotevant and McRoy 1998; Sykes 2000) and the agency may need to provide careful mediation in order to smooth out misunderstandings.

Both adoptive and birth families may need support in planning and maintaining indirect contact (Milham et al. 1986). Adoptive parents may find writing letters to birth parents about an adopted child's progress challenging or they may want advice about how to share a birth relative's letter with their adopted child. All parties may feel disappointed or disturbed by the content of letters or cards and mediation may be required to achieve more satisfactory exchanges.

One problem that is often encountered in post box contact is the non-response of birth parents to requests for letters. Some birth parents do not value themselves as a potential resource for their adopted child, for example, as a source of information, or they may be impeded by feelings of guilt, anger, inadequacy or practical barriers. They may need personal support and practical help in overcoming these difficulties.

If such approaches are unsuccessful, adopted children may need help in understanding and coming to terms with this aspect of their birth parents' behaviour.

Model of adoption support – supporting in face-to-face contact

Some agencies provide an enhanced service to facilitate in face-to-face contact which include arranging meetings to discuss difficulties, offering emotional or practical support to adopters or birth parents around contact issues such as writing letters, making phone calls, or keeping adopters informed of birth parents' whereabouts or wellbeing. Such support has been shown to be highly valued by adoptive and birth families (Neil 2002).

Case example – supporting in face-to-face contact

Harry, a 9-year-old boy, was not truly settling into his adoptive family despite having been there for five years. He was aggressive and non-accepting towards his adoptive mother. Therapeutic work, which included going over his story, looking at the photographs of his birth family and role-playing questions to the birth family, still did not satisfy his need to have his questions answered and to confirm that his mother was well. It was not felt helpful for him to have face-to-face contact. Instead it was suggested that a video of his birth mother answering his questions could be made. This required a lot of careful preparation and support of his birth mother and the adoptive parents. For the boy, when he watched the video, the reality of seeing his birth mother, hearing her voice talking to him, using his name and answering his questions had a striking impact. He was finally able to believe that she wanted him to be in his adoptive family as she could not care for him herself and that she wanted him to be happy

---

Face-to-face contact

Contact venue

A good quality venue is essential, as this will convey positive messages to children and adults about the value of the contact. Venues should also be suitable for the child's age, interests and wishes and suitable for the level of monitoring and confidentiality. Adopted children's needs and wishes regarding venue will change as they grow older (Macaskill 2002).

Making the arrangements

For younger adopted children where contact is relatively straightforward, research indicates that agencies should aim to support adoptive and birth families where desired and/or necessary, but should be mindful of need not to undermine people's confidence in taking control of arrangements themselves where they want to and feel able to. On the whole, self-sustaining arrangements appeared to be more robust and satisfying for all concerned (Neil 2002). However, families of later placed adopted children have underlined the critical importance of a professional support service underpinning contact arrangements (Rushton and Dance 2003). In these cases, contact could involve intricate and highly charged relationships and the potential for conflict was high. Families greatly welcomed the availability of an intermediary and when there were difficulties, this made it more likely that the contact would continue.

Supporting adopted children

For younger adopted children, it is generally felt preferable for the adoptive parents to support the child during meetings, providing security and a clear message about who is the primary parent (Neil 2002). However, teenagers who are settled in their placements have expressed the preference of having a more neutral person to accompany them. Many found the emotional turmoil of being in the presence of both families to be very disturbing (Dance and Rushton 2005a). Relinking with birth families evokes memories and responses for the adopted child. This can lead to the adopted child being distressed or upset following contact, or presenting with behaviour which adoptive parents find challenging or oppositional. Adoptive parents may need help to develop strategies for reducing the impact of the contact arrangements, or the arrangements themselves may need adjustment.

Supporting adopters and special guardians

A study of 76 families with 106 adopted children showed that contact could generate considerable emotional turmoil in the adults (Macaskill 2002). It could be a trigger for the pain associated with infertility, or abuse in their own childhood, or there could be distress caused by the loss and grief of the birth parent. Adoptive parents who felt unsupported by their agencies reported feelings of isolation and of having been let down. There were also cases of important contact disintegrating after the order was made, due to the lack of professional support. Black and Asian adoptive families, in the same study, felt more comfortable if their social worker's background was similar to their own. Adoptive families wished for a proactive rather than a reactive service. Agencies should be sensitive to all of these issues when planning post-placement contact.

When contact is an area of concern for adoptive parents, where it is presenting difficulties for the adopted child or the birth family, or when the courts have ordered contact but the contact arrangements are proving problematic, further mediation and negotiation may be required. Potentially difficult contact needs to be firmly controlled to prevent adopted children experiencing further harm, and there will be situations where it is beneficial to the child to cease contact (Macaskill 2002; Sinclair et al. 2004b).

Children who are subject to special guardianship are more likely to have contact with parents and other family members. Where a child is cared for by special guardians who are members of the extended family, the emotional context of contact is likely to be particularly complex, so appropriate support will be essential. Until they have experienced them, prospective carers are likely to underestimate the difficulty of managing contact in such a context. Workers may therefore need to be both proactive and sensitive in encouraging carers to accept support.

Financial support

There may be considerable resource implications in some face-to-face contact arrangements and there is a risk that inadequate contact arrangements are made because an adoptive family's finances are limited (Scott and Lindsey 2003). Agencies should underpin contact plans with adequate financial support wherever possible.

Contact with birth siblings

Face-to-face contact with birth siblings forms a significant proportion of face-to-face contact arrangements, and research suggests that the majority of such arrangements work well and can be more straightforward than contact with birth parents (Macaskill 2002; Rushton et al. 2001). However, complexities can arise over time and on occasions, the meetings can evoke painful memories of unresolved trauma. Previous negative behaviour patterns between siblings can also re-emerge and should be carefully managed. Careful planning is therefore required, with clear expectations about who, where and how often and fully negotiated written agreements. A third party appointed to provide ongoing mediation and adjustments may be helpful, along with a review system to ensure that the plan is updated and satisfactory.

Search and reunion with older adopted children and young people

For young people who have not had face-to-face contact with their birth relatives over the years, the desire to make personal contact can become very strong. Agencies may not support a young person under the age of 18 in searching for birth relatives without the consent of their parents. Sometimes, however, parents may feel that a supported search, preceded by counselling, is the best way forward. Such counselling will require a carefully judged and sensitive approach. In some cases, the young person might simply need a chance to talk through thoughts and feelings about birth family members, the circumstances of the adoption, hopes and fears regarding reunion and so on. In others, the provision of further information from the file might be sufficient for the time being.

When the desire to search for relatives remains paramount, careful counselling and support is required for all parties, including the birth relatives. Wherever possible, it is helpful to work in partnership with adoptive parents and the young person together. Ideally, there should be a gradual process of information gathering, talking thorough the potential scenarios and pitfalls that may be encountered and weighing up the benefits and risks of proceeding further. If the social worker is able to act as an intermediary, all parties can be better prepared for the realities of the situation prior to a meeting. However, it also has to be remembered that young people may act independently in making contact and further support may be required by all parties to deal with the impact of this.

Although it is to be hoped that adoptive parents will have shared background information appropriately and talked openly about adoption issues, there are a small number of cases in which this will not have happened and the young person's knowledge is very limited. A young person might seek information independently, with or without a view to searching for relatives. Agencies should have a clearly defined policy for such cases. They will need to bear in mind not only the status of the young person as a minor and the parental responsibility of the adoptive parents, but also the capacity of the young person to search independently and the physical and emotional risk that this could entail.

Sometimes, there are particular circumstances that have to be taken into account. For example, a young person might have become estranged from their adoptive family and wish for contact with birth family members. Each situation will be unique and there may be a case for flexibility in an agency's policies and procedures. Some agencies have an Ethical Advisory Forum where dilemmas can be discussed and a decision reached within a broad range of expertise and advice (Feast 2003).

Annex I

Chart of information gathered by use of evidence-based assessment tools in assessing adoption support needs using domains and dimensions of the *Assessment Framework*

For references for assessment tools see end of charts. A range of evidence based assessment tools are referred to throughout this book. This chart indicates the information which the specific assessment tools help to gather under the domains and dimensions of the *Assessment Framework*.

Child's Developmental Needs Domain of the Assessment Framework

Assessment Tools	Health *Physical and mental well-being of child*	Education *Cognitive development and educational needs*	Emotional and behavioural development *Feelings and responses of child toward others*	Identity *Child's sense of self and self-esteem*	Family and social relationships *Development of relationships and empathy*	Social presentation *Child's understanding of how to present self in outside world*	Self-care skills *Child's practical, emotional and communication skills*
Strengths and Difficulties Questionnaires **	Gives screening information about emotional and behavioural problems and needs in children and young people aged 3–16. Can show how problems affecting child's schooling are impacting on and impacted by child's health. D	Gives information about the child's adjustment at school and difficulties in learning. It indicates whether there is a need for a specialist assessment. D	For children and young people 3–16, screens for prosocial behaviour, hyperactivity, emotional, conduct (behavioural) and peer relationship problems at home and at school. D	Looks at children's relationships with peers, their friendships, and leisure activities and how they are perceived at home and at school. D	Looks at children's relationships with peers, their friendships and leisure activities and how they are perceived at home and at school. D	Looks at impact of strengths and difficulties on learning, relationships and what impacts on this aspect of child development. D	D
Parenting Daily Hassles Scale			May provide cues to emotional and behavioural difficulties and description of strengths and problems encountered. D	Looks at quality of relationships between child and brothers and sisters. D		D	D
Home Conditions Scale							Assesses state of child's own room and belongings. O

Adult Wellbeing Scale				D			
Adolescent Wellbeing Scale **		Discussion of impact of young person's emotional state on his or her learning and relationships at school. D	Screens for depression. Impact of difficulties encountered by a young person on his or her friendships, home life and leisure activities. D		Helps identify adopted young person's own perceptions of family and social relationships and impact of adolescent's emotional state. D		Impact of recent life events on child's development. D
Recent Life Events Questionnaire	Illness and recent hospitalisation of child. D	Change of school or home. D	Impact of recent events on child's development. D	Discussion of impact of recent life events on child's development. D	Impact of recent life events on child's development. D	Impact of recent events on child's development. D	Impact of recent life events on child's development. D
Family Activity Scale	Impact of illness or disability on family activity. D			Picks up on involvement in independent activities. D	Child's participation in child-centred family activity and child's independent activities. D	How child manages self-presentation in independent activities. D	
Alcohol Scale	Discussion may reveal neglect, lack of supervision that is leading to child's impairment. D						

Child's Developmental Needs Domain of the Assessment Framework

Assessment Tools	Health *Physical and mental well-being of child*	Education *Cognitive development and educational needs*	Emotional and behavioural development *Feelings and responses of child toward others*	Identity *Child's sense of self and self-esteem*	Family and social relationships *Development of relationships and empathy*	Social presentation *Child's understanding of how to present self in outside world*	Self-care skills *Child's practical, emotional and communication skills*
Sheridan Charts **	Maps developmental progress of infants and young children and helps indicate need for assessment of children's cognitive development when placed and in tracking their progress during placement. **D**	Maps developmental progress of infants and young children and helps establish need for assessment of cognitive development when placed and in tracking progress during placement. **D**					
HOME Inventory	Through the exploration of events of the day a good picture emerges of children's physical and mental well-being and their development. Contacts with medical services. **O + R**	Assesses the learning environment provided for children at home and how they are responding and, with older children, how they are responding at school. **O + R**	Child's responses to caregiving by care-givers and to daily events. Observation of emotional states, how distress is managed and the presence of anxiety, mood difficulties and opposition/defiance problems. **O + R**	Child's assertiveness and confidence in interactions at home. Allows observation of the environment of encouragement, individuality and a sense of belonging and the child's responses. **O + R**	Gathers information about the nature and quality of parent–child interactions and involvement and the child's contact with other family members and extended family. **O + R**	How child is responding to opportunities for social contact and leisure opportunities available for the child. Observed social skills. **O + R**	Systematically explores range of self-care skills, e.g. washing, dressing, mealtimes, getting to school, and encouragement given to develop self-care skills and adaptation to child's specific needs. **O + R**

Family Assessment	Through observation of a child during a *Family Assessment* a good picture emerges of the child's physical and mental well-being and his or her development. **O + R**	Explores key factors affecting the child's cognitive development and education, including stimulation and encouragement, parent–child relationships and communication in the family. **O + R**	Looks at nature of attachment in family, including pattern of care-seeking behaviour of the adopted child, how emotions are expressed/responded to and difficulties in child's emotional and behavioural development. **O + R**	*Family Identity* can help assess how adopted child is developing as an individual, the child's self-assertiveness and autonomy, the degree of emotional involvement and sense of 'together-ness' as an adoptive family. **O + R**	Strengths and difficulties in child's relationships with family, including with parents, brothers and sisters, and extended family and birth and foster families. **O + R**	Helps identify how the child is adapting to the family as he or she settles in and becomes a member of the family and the emergence of self-presentation and the nature of social relationships. **O + R**	Through observation and in the evaluation of parenting a picture of the development of the child's self-care skills emerges. **O + R**
Fahlberg's Observation Checklists			Provide a useful guide to assessing attachment behaviours (and care-givers' responses) for children from infancy to adolescence.				
In My Shoes (IMS) **	Has a module for talking about and gaining an understanding of children's experiences of pain, including accidents, illness, hospital treatment, abuse and emotional pain. **O + D**	Has a set of school scenes and other tools to help children talk about their school experience, including their thoughts and their feelings about lessons, teachers, peers, playtime, homework. **O + D**	Allows worker to explore with children their emotional and behavioural responses to different, scenes, living and other settings and people and how they understand and experience different aspects of their lives. **O + D**	Is used interactively with children to build up a picture of them and their world and their emotional responses to things that have happened to them and the people in their lives. Pictures generated from the interview can be printed out. **O + D**	Exploring the relationship between children's emotions and the places and people in their lives (e.g. family, school, park, previous and future families etc.). **O + D**	Looking at how children see themselves fitting in the contexts in which they live and their understanding of how they present themselves and how others see them. **O + D**	Gathering a picture of children's self-care skills in different settings, assistance to gain self-care skills and about learning to look after themselves. **O + D**

1

O = information that may be revealed by observation when using assessment tools

R = information that is explored in interview schedules

D = information that may be revealed by discussion of specific items in assessment tools. Discussion focuses on the meaning of particular scores or items to person, and explores how that factor affects, or is affected by aspects of child's developmental needs, parenting capacity and/or family and environmental factors

** = key tool for assessing dimensions in the domain

Parenting Capacity Domain of the Assessment Framework

Assessment Tools	Basic care *Providing for child's physical needs*	Ensuring safety *Ensuring child protected from harm and danger*	Emotional warmth *Ensuring child's emotional needs are met*	Stimulation *Promoting child's learning and intellectual development*	Guidance and boundaries *Enabling child to regulate their own emotions and behaviour*	Stability *Providing stable environment for developing attachments*
Strengths and Difficulties Questionnaires	D	D	D	D	D	D
Parenting Daily Hassles (PDH) Scale **	Discussion of PDH Scale may reveal strengths and difficulties in all areas of parenting including basic care. D	Discussion may raise issues regarding ensuring safety. D	Strengths and difficulties in relation to emotional warmth may arise from discussion. D	Allows for discussion of how provide learning opportunities for child and encouragement, reassurance and praise. D	Looks at current areas of difficulty parents may be facing in managing a child's behaviour. D	Discussion of PDH Scale can focus whether parents need support in providing a stable environment for the child. D
Home Conditions Scale **	Hygiene relevant to health.	Tour of home may identify dangers or risks to child's safety. O				
Adult Wellbeing Scale	Discussion of impact parental state on all aspects of parenting. D	Impact of parental outwards directed hostility on ensuring safety. D	Impact of parental outwards directed hostility or depression on emotional warmth. D	Parental depression may be relevant due to impact on stimulation. D	Parental depression and anxiety may impact on guidance and boundaries. D	Impact of parental hostility, anxiety and/or depression on stability. D

Adolescent Wellbeing Scale	Discussion of impact on child care. D	Discussion of parental response to what is reported by young person. D			Discussion of parental response to what is reported by young person. D
Recent Life Events Questionnaire		Discussion of impact on child care. D		Discussion of impact on child care. D	Changes of partners and house moves. D
Family Activity Scale	Can explore whether there is adequate supervision. D	Identifies child-centred family activities and support for independent activity. D	Identifies child-centred family activities and support for independent activity.		
Alcohol Scale	Discussion of impact of alcohol misuse on basic care. D	Looking at effect of alcohol misuse on providing emotional warmth. D	Exploring if alcohol misuse affects parents' capacity to offer child learning opportunities, praise etc. D	Discussion of impact of alcohol misuse on giving children appropriate guidance and boundaries. D	Discussion of impact of alcohol misuse stability of the home environment and caregiving offered. D
Sheridan Charts	Discussion of parental response to what is reported about child's health and development. D	Information given about by parents about play and social behaviour. D	Discussion about parents report on children's physical and social development. D	Discussion about how parents mange child's developing social behaviour and play. D	Discussion of parents' response to child's relationships with them and other family members. D

Parenting Capacity Domain of the Assessment Framework

Assessment Tools	Basic care *Providing for child's physical needs*	Ensuring safety *Ensuring child protected from harm and danger*	Emotional warmth *Ensuring child's emotional needs are met*	Stimulation *Promoting child's learning and intellectual development*	Guidance and boundaries *Enabling child to regulate their own emotions and behaviour*	Stability *Providing stable environment for developing attachments*
HOME Inventory **	Gives an opportunity to assess in detail whether a child's basic care needs are being met and to identify any difficulties adoptive parents may be having in adapting to a child's extra needs.	Looks at issues of safety in the child's home environment.	Specifically addresses emotional sensitivity and responsivity of the care giver towards the child and helps to locate the exact nature of any difficulties parents are experiencing in day-to-day care.	Covers adoptive parents' provision of stimulation, support, and opportunities for play and learning that support cognitive development of adopted child. Includes provision of play and learning materials, language, academic stimulation and encouragement of play and learning.	Specifically addresses modelling by parents, the use of boundaries in parent–child relationships, how parents set limits for children and discipline them, how they encourage the development of socially responsible and mature behaviour.	Provides information about changes child's circumstances and relationships; and about parental responsivity and acceptance of child and the emotional climate.
	O + R	O + R	O + R	O + R	O + R	O + R
Family Assessment **	*Parenting* component explores the way the family manages basic care tasks and responds to the changing needs of the child.	*Parenting* helps to highlight strengths and difficulties in ensuring safety, looking at the nature of attachments and the protection, care and management of children.	Helps to assess nature of attachments, parent–child and other family relationships, how feelings are expressed and responded to, whether relationships are supported and appreciative and the level of emotional involvement.	Explores how adoptive parents promote a child's development through stimulation, emotional warmth and praise.	Looks at strengths and difficulties parents have in providing guidance, boundary setting, protection and their expectations of the children, and associated aspects of family life, including decision-making, problem solving and the management of conflicts.	Explores caregiving and the nature of the attachments and the parent–child relationship and how feelings are expressed and responded to in the family.
	O + R	O + R	O + R	O + R	O + R	O + R

	Basic care	Ensuring safety	Emotional warmth	Stimulation	Guidance and boundaries	Attachments
Fahlberg's Observation Checklists		Gives information about parents' sensitivity to child's needs for ensuring safety. O + D	Useful guide to child's attachment behaviours level of responsiveness and sensitivity shown by the caregiver. O + D	Provides information about stimulation and parents' responsiveness towards child. O + D		Explores level of responsiveness and sensitivity of care-giver, helps identify strengths and areas where support may be useful. O + D
In My Shoes	Provides information about basic care provided for a child and child's response. O + D	Helps gain picture of how far child is kept safe and how far child understands issues of safety. O + D	Gain picture of child's view of emotional warmth provided by carers and child's response to that. O + D	Child's report on assistance given by carers with educational tasks and opportunities to develop cognitive and social skills. O + D	Explore guidance and boundaries provided by carers from child's perspective, including abusive or neglectful parenting. O + D	Gather picture of carers capacity to help child build attachments with family members and child's view of how secure their place in the family feels. O + D

Family and Environmental Factors Domain of the Assessment Framework

Assessment Tools	Family history and functioning *Significant family history, individual wellbeing and family functioning*	Wider family *Role and importance of wider family, including adopted child's birth family*	Housing *Appropriateness of accommodation to needs of child, family and other resident members*	Employment *Pattern of employment and impact on child and family members' relationship with child*	Income *Sufficiency of income to meet family needs and available resources*	Family's social integration *Integration with neighbourhood and community; peer groups, friendships and social networks*	Community resources *Availability, accessibility and standard of facilities and services available in community*
Strengths and Difficulties Questionnaires	Discussion may reveal parental mental health issues or difficulties in family functioning. D						
Parenting Daily Hassles Scale	Helpful in identifying aspects of care that may put extra strain on adoptive parents. D	Helpful in identifying aspects of contact with wider family that may be difficult. D					
Home Conditions Scale **			Addresses standards of cleanliness.				
Adult Wellbeing Scale **	Explores how an adult is feeling in terms of depression, anxiety and irritability and can indicate when professional help may be beneficial. D						
Adolescent Wellbeing Scale							

Recent Life Events Questionnaire **	Impact of illness and death on family functioning. D	Impact of illness and death, recent moves and other life events on wider family. D	Effect of recent house moves; can be a major life event for family members. D	Impact of employment difficulties on parents and children. D	Effect of financial difficulties family members. D	Support from or conflicts with neighbours. D	
Family Activity Scale	Social activities of family explored. D		Discussion may reveal effects of housing on joint activities families can do together. D	May reveal adverse effects of employment problems on joint family activities. D	Impact of financial difficulties on joint family activities. D		Explores family's child-centred use of community facilities and resources in terms of leisure. D
Alcohol Scale **	Impact on health. Valuable way of exploring any potential difficulties with alcohol use. D			Impact on employment. D	Impact on income. D	Social use of alcohol and family's social integration. Impact of any misuse on relationships with neighbours and friends. D	
Sheridan Charts							
HOME Inventory **	Information on parental mental health and family functioning may be observed or reported. O + R	Looks at the child's contact and relationship with members of the wider family. O + R	Provides information on housing as part of an assessment of the adopted child's home environment. Includes context of home in neighbourhood. O + R	A *HOME Inventory* conducted with birth parent or foster carer can help predict levels of care on adopted child is likely to need and the potential impact on the employment pattern of the adoptive parents. O + R		Family's contact with friends and neighbours. O + R	Family's use of community resources or need for access to additional resources or facilities may be reported. O + R

Family and Environmental Factors Domain of the Assessment Framework

Assessment Tools	Family history and functioning	Wider family	Housing	Employment	Income	Family's social integration	Community resources
	Significant family history, individual wellbeing and family functioning	*Role and importance of wider family, including adopted child's birth family*	*Appropriateness of accommodation to needs of child, family and other resident members*	*Pattern of employment and impact on child and family members' relationship with child*	*Sufficiency of income to meet family needs and available resources*	*Integration with neighbourhood and community; peer groups, friendships and social networks*	*Availability, accessibility and standard of facilities and services available in community*
Family Assessment ******	Looks at crucial everyday inter-actions with which families may need support, including decision making, problem solving, managing conflict, family communi-cation and how feelings are expressed and responded to, family alliances and family identity. *Family history* systematically explores the mean-ing and impact of past significant events and relationships and can help identify unresolved issues from the past.	Explores the family's relationships with the wider family. *Mapping the problem* helps identify resources and areas of difficulty in wider adopted family, and regarding contact with birth family and significant others.	Observation and discussion of housing needs possible as part of *Family Assessment* carried out in home.	Information may be revealed during discussion in *Family* Assessment.	Information may be revealed during discussion in *Family* Assessment.	Family's relation-ships with the wider family and commun-ity gives picture of strengths and difficulties in family's relation-ships with the wider family and community, includ-ing whether the adoptive parents have been able to maintain their friendships and support networks.	Family's use of community resources or need for access to additional resources or facilities may be reported.
O + R	**O + R**	**O + R**	**O + D**	**O + D**	**O + D**	**R**	**R**

Fahlberg's Observation Checklists							
In My Shoes (IMS)	Explores children's experience of family relationships and relates their thoughts, wishes and feelings. O + D	Enables children to communicate about their birth family, wider adoptive family and adoptive family and their contact with each. O + D	IMS can be used to help children to talk about the houses they have lived in, with whom etc. O + D	Discussion of family life using IMS can include employment of adoptive parents and impact on child. O + D	Issues and concerns about income may be revealed through use of IMS with a child.	Exploration of child and family's wider social networks facilitated through IMS including gauging child's related feelings. O + D	Child's (and family's) involvement with community resources can be tracked using IMS.
Attachment Style Interview for Adoption and Fostering	Explores adopters' attachment styles and use of support offered by their significantly close people in their lives. R + O	Assists in assessing support available to adopters in the wider family and their views about other people and using support. R + O				Gives information about adopters' involvement with and attitude towards immediate and wider family network and others. R + O	May give information about adopters' involvement with community resources and their use and views about using them for support. R + O

References for assessment tools

Further information about many of the assessment tools discussed in the chart can be found on www.childandfamilytraining.org.uk.

The Family Pack of Questionnaires and Scales: Department of Health, Cox A and Bentovim A (2000) *The Family Pack of Questionnaires and Scales.* The Stationery Office, London.

The HOME Inventory: Cox A and Walker S (2002) *The HOME Inventory.* Child and Family Training, London.

The Family Assessment: Assessment of Family Competence, Strengths and Difficulties: Bentovim A and Bingley Miller L (2001) *The Family Assessment.* Child and Family Training, London.

Chart Illustrating the Development Progress of Infants and Young Children: Sheridan M, in Department of Health (2000) *Assessing Children in Need and their Families: Practice Guidance.* The Stationery Office, London.

Observation Checklists: Fahlberg V (1994) *A Child's Journey through Placement,* BAAF, London.

In My Shoes: Calam RM, Cox AD, Glasgow DV, Jimmieson P and Groth Larsen S (2000) Assessment and therapy with children: Can computers help? *Child Clinical Psychology and Psychiatry* **5(3)**: 329–43.

Attachment Style Interview: Bifulco A, Moran P, Ball C and Bernazzani O (2002a) Adult Attachment Style I: Its relationship to clinical depression. *Social Psychiatry and Psychiatric Epidemiology* **37**: 50–9. and Bifulco A, Moran P, Ball C and Lillie A (2002b) Adult Attachment Style II: Its relationship to psychosocial depressive-vulnerability. *Social Psychiatry and Psychiatric Epidemiology* **37**: 60–7.

Bibliography

Adoption UK (2000) *It's a Piece of Cake? A new parent support programme developed by adopters for adopters*. Adoption UK, Daventry.

Ainsworth MDS, Blehar M, Walters E and Wall S (1978) *Patterns of Attachment: A psychological study of the strange situation*. Lawrence Erlbaum, Hillsdale, NJ.

Archer C (2000a) *First Steps in Parenting the Child Who Hurts*. Jessica Kingsley, London.

Archer C (2000b) *Next Steps in Parenting the Child Who Hurts*. Jessica Kingsley, London.

Archer C and Burnell A (2003) *Trauma, Attachment and Family Permanence*. Jessica Kingsley, London.

Archer C and Gordon C (2004) Parenting mentoring: An innovative approach to adoption support. *Adoption and Fostering* **(28)**4: 27–38.

Argent H (1996) *Post Adoption Services for Children with Disabilities (Practice Paper)*. Post Adoption Centre, London.

Argent H (1997) *Taking Extra Care*. BAAF, London.

Argent H (1998) *Whatever Happened to Adam?* BAAF, London.

Argent H (ed.) (2003b) *Models of Adoption Support: What works and what doesn't*. BAAF, London.

Argent H (2003a) Adoption support for disabled children and their families. In Argent H (ed.) *Models of Adoption Support*. BAAF, London.

Argent H and Kerrane A (1997) *Taking Extra Care: Shared, respite and permanent care for children with disabilities*. BAAF, London.

BAAF (2006) Attachment Disorders, their Assessment and Intervention/Treatment: Position Statement 4. BAAF, London.

Ball C (2005) The Adoption and Children Act 2002: A critical examination. *Adoption and Fostering* **29(2)**: 6–17.

Beckett C, Castle J, Groothues C, O'Connor J, Rutter M and the English and Romanian Study Team (2003) Health problems in children adopted from Romania: Association with duration of deprivation and behavioural problems. *Adoption and Fostering* **27(4)**: 19–29.

Beek M (1999) *Parenting children with attachment difficulties: Views of adoptive parents and implications for post-adoption services. Adoption and Fostering* **23(1)**: 16–23.

Beek M and Schofield G (2004a) Providing a secure base: Tuning in to children with severe learning difficulties in long-term foster care. *Adoption and Fostering* **28(2)**: 8–19.

Beek M and Schofield G (2004b) *Providing a Secure Base in Long-term Foster Care*. BAAF, London.

Bentovim A (2002) Preventing sexually abused young people from becoming abusers, and treating the victimization experiences of young people who offend sexually. *Child Abuse and Neglect* **26(67)**: 661–78.

Bentovim A (2006) Therapeutic interventions with children who have experienced sexual and physical abuse in the UK. In McAuley C, Pecora C and Rose W (eds) *Enhancing the*

Wellbeing of Children and Families through Effective Interventions. Jessica Kingsley, London.

Bentovim A and Bingley Miller L (2001) *The Family Assessment: Assessment of family competence, strengths and difficulties.* Child and Family Training, London.

Betts B and Ahmad A (2003) *My Life Story (CD-Rom).* BAAF, London.

Bifulco A, Moran P, Ball C and Bernazzani O (2002a) Adult Attachment Style I: Its relationship to clinical depression. *Social Psychiatry and Psychiatric Epidemiology* 37: 50–9.

Bifulco A, Moran P, Ball C and Lillie A (2002b) Adult Attachment Style II: Its relationship to psychosocial depressive-vulnerability. *Social Psychiatry and Psychiatric Epidemiology* 37: 60–7.

Birleson P (1980) The validity of depressive disorder in childhood and the development of a self-rating scale: A research report. *Journal of Child Psychology and Psychiatry* 22: 73–88.

Borland M, O'Hara G and Triseliotis J (1991) Permanent outcomes for children with special needs. *Adoption and Fostering* 15(2): 18–28.

Bowlby J (1969) *Attachment.* Vol. 1 of *Attachment and Loss.* Penguin, Harmondsworth.

Bowlby J (1973) *Separation: Anxiety and anger.* Vol. 2 of *Attachment and Loss.* Penguin, Harmondsworth.

British Association for Adoption and Fostering (1999) *Contact in Permanent Placement: Guidance for local authorities in England and Wales and Scotland.* BAAF, London.

British Association for Adoption and Fostering (2006) *Attachment Disorders, their Assessment and Intervention/Treatment.* Position Statement. BAAF, London.

Broad B (2001) Kinship care: Supporting children in placements with extended family and friends. *Adoption and Fostering* 25(2): 33–41.

Broad B and Skinner A (2005) *Relative Benefits: Placing children in kinship care.* BAAF, London.

Brodzinsky DM (1987) Adjustment to adoption: A psychosocial perspective. *Clinical Psychological Review* 7: 25–47.

Brodzinsky DM (1990) A stress and coping model of adoption adjustment. In Brodzinsky DM and Schechter MD (eds) *The Psychology of Adoption.* Oxford University Press, New York.

Brodzinsky DM, Smith DW and Brodzinsky AB (1998) *Children's Adjustment to Adoption: Developmental and clinical issues.* Sage, Thousand Oaks, CA.

Brugha T, Bebington P, Tennant C and Hurry J (1985) The list of threatening experiences: A subset of 12 life events categories with considerable long-term contextual threat. *Psychological Medicine* 15: 189–94.

Burnell A (2003) Assessment: A multidisciplinary approach. In Archer C and Burnell A (eds) *Trauma, Attachment and Family Permanence.* Jessica Kingsley, London.

Byrne S and Chambers L (1997a) *Living with a New Family: Nadia and Rashid's story.* BAAF, London.

Byrne S and Chambers L (1997b) *Belonging Doesn't Mean Forgetting: Nathan's story.* BAAF, London.

Byrne S and Chambers L (1999) *Joining Together: Jo's story.* BAAF, London.

Cairns K (2001) The effects of trauma on childhood learning. In Jackson S (ed.) *Nobody Ever Told Us School Mattered.* BAAF, London.

Cairns K (2002) *Attachment, Trauma and Resilience.* BAAF, London.

Calam RM, Cox AD, Glasgow DV, Jimmieson P and Groth Larsen S (2000) Assessment and therapy with children: Can computers help? *Child Clinical Psychology and Psychiatry* 5(3): 329–43.

Camis J (2001) *My Life and Me.* BAAF, London.

Chamberlain K and Horne J (2003) Understanding normality in adoptive family life: The role of peer group support. In Argent H (ed.) *Models of Adoption Support.* BAAF, London.

Charlton L, Crank M, Kansara K and Oliver C (1998) *Still Screaming: Birth parents compulsorily separated from their children.* After Adoption, Manchester.

Chennells P and Morrison M (1998) *Talking about Adoption.* BAAF, London.

Clapton G (2000) Perceptions of fatherhood: Birth fathers and their adoption experiences. *Adoption and Fostering* **24(3)**: 69–70.

Cleaver H (2003) *Assessing Children's Needs and Circumstances: The impact of the Assessment Framework. Summary and recommendations.* Department of Health, London.

Cleaver H, Unel I and Aldgate A (1999) *Children's Needs and Parenting Capacity: The impact of parental mental illness, problem alcohol and drug use and domestic violence on children's behaviour.* The Stationery Office, London.

Cooper A (2005) Surface and depth in the Victoria Climbie Report. *Child and Family Social Work* **10(1)**: 1–9.

Cousins J (2003) Are we missing the match? Rethinking adopter assessment and child profiling. *Adoption and Fostering* **27(4)**: 7–18.

Cousins J (2006) Every Child is Special – placing disabled children for permenance. BAAF, London.

Cox A and Walker S (2002) *The HOME Inventory.* Child and Family Training, London.

Dance C and Rushton A (2005a) Joining a new family: The views and experiences of young people placed with permanent families during middle childhood. *Adoption and Fostering* **29(1)**: 18–28.

Dance C and Rushton A (2005b) *Predictors of outcomes for unrelated adoptive placements made during middle childhood. Child and Family Social Work* **10(4)**: 269–80.

Davie C, Hutt S, Vincent E and Mason M (1984) *The Young Child at Home.* NFER-Nelson, Windsor.

Department for Education and Skills (2002) *Code of Practice for Special Educational Needs.* HMSO, London.

Department for Education and Skills (2003a) *Every Child Matters.* The Stationery Office, London.

Department for Education and Skills (2003b) *Statistics of Education: Children Looked After in England: 2002–2003.* National Statistics Bulletin, Issue no. 06/03. The Stationery Office, London.

Department for Education and Skills (2003c) *Statistics of Education: Children Looked After in England: 2002–2003.* National Statistics Bulletin, Issue no. 07/03. The Stationery Office, London.

Department for Education and Skills (2005a) *Adoption Support Services Regulations.* DfES, London.

Department for Education and Skills (2005b) *Practice Guidance on Assessing the Support Needs of Adoptive Families.* DfES, London.

Department for Education and Skills (2005c) *The Adoption Agencies Regulations 2005, SI 389.* The Stationery Office, London.

Department for Education and Skills (2006) *Practice Guidance on Assessing Adopters.* DfES, London.

Department of Health (1999a) *Promoting Health for Looked After Children: A guide to healthcare planning assessment and monitoring.* Consultation document. HMSO, London.

Department of Health (1999b) *The Education of Young People in Public Care.* HMSO, London.

Department of Health (2000a) *Assessing Children in Need and their Families: Practice guidance.* The Stationery Office, London.

Department of Health (2000b) *Integrated Children's System: Working with children in need and their families.* Draft Consultation Document. Department of Health, London.

Department of Health (2002a) *Promoting the Health of Looked After Children.* HMSO, London.

Department of Health (2002b) *Providing Effective Adoption Support*. The Stationery Office, London.

Department of Health, Cox A and Bentovim A (2000a) *The Family Pack of Questionnaires and Scales*. The Stationery Office, London.

Department of Health, Department for Education and Employment, and Home Office (2000b) *Framework for the Assessment of Children in Need and their Families*. The Stationery Office, London.

Department of Health, Home Office and Department for Education and Skills (2006) *Working Together to Safeguard Children: A guide to inter-agency working to safeguard and promote the welfare of children*. Department of Health, London.

Dozier M (2003) Attachment-based treatment for vulnerable children. *Attachment and Human Development* **5(3)**: 223–44.

Dozier M, Stovall KC and Albus KE (1998) Enhancing sensitivity to attachment issues among caregivers of foster infants. In Cicetti D and Toth SI (eds) *Rochester Symposium on Developmental Psychopathology: Developmental approaches to prevention and intervention*. University of Rochester Press, Rochester, NY.

Duck M (2003) Working with black adopted children and their families. In Argent H (ed.) *Models of Adoption Support*. BAAF, London.

Eccles S (2003) Youth work with adopted children and young people. In Argent H (ed.) *Models of Adoption Support*. BAAF, London.

Fahlberg V (1994) *A Child's Journey through Placement*. BAAF, London.

Farina L, Leifer M and Chasnoff I (2004) Attachment and behavioural difficulties in internationally adopted Russian children. *Adoption and Fostering* **28(2)**: 38–49.

Feast J (2003) Adoption support services for adults. In Argent H (ed.) *Models of Adoption Support*. BAAF, London.

Feast J and Howe D (2003) Talking and telling. In Douglas A and Philpot T (eds) *Adoption: Changing families, changing times*. Routledge, London.

Firth H and Fletcher B (2001) Developing equal chances. In Jackson S (ed.) *Nobody Ever Told Us School Mattered*. BAAF, London.

Fletcher-Campbell F (2001) Current educational initiatives. In Jackson S (ed.) *Nobody Ever Told Us School Mattered*. BAAF, London.

Foxon J (2001) *Nutmeg Gets Adopted*. BAAF, London.

Fratter J, Rowe J, Sapsford D and Thoburn J (1991) *Permanent Family Placement: A decade of experience*. BAAF, London.

Gilkes L and Klimes I (2003) Parenting skills for adoptive parents. *Adoption and Fostering* **27(1)**: 19–25.

Gilligan R (2000) *Promoting Resilience*. BAAF, London.

Glaser D (2000) Child abuse and neglect and the brain – A review. *Journal of Child Psychology and Psychiatry* **41(1)**: 97–116.

Golding K (2003) Helping foster carers, helping children: Using attachment theory to guide practice. *Adoption and Fostering* **27(2)**: 64–73.

Goodman R (1997) The Strengths and Difficulties Questionnaire: A research note. *Journal of Child Psychology and Psychiatry* **35(5)**: 581–6.

Gordon C (2003) Holding the fort. In Archer C and Burnell A (eds) *Trauma, Attachment and Family Permanence*. Jessica Kingsley, London.

Grant A (1995) The role of the medical adviser. In Turnpenny P (ed.) *Secrets in the Genes*. BAAF, London.

Greenmile L (2003) 'A Hard Day's Night'. A parent's perspective. In Archer C and Burnell A (eds) *Trauma, Attachment and Family Permanence*. Jessica Kingsley, London.

Greenwood S and Forster S (undated) *Tell Me Who I am: Young people talk about adoption*. After Adoption, Manchester.

Grotevant HD and McRoy RG (1998) *Openness in Adoption: Exploring family connections.* Sage, Thousand Oaks, CA.

Harnott C and Robertson R (1999) Intercountry adoption: Implications for adoption agencies and medical advisers. *Adoption and Fostering* **23(4)**: 26–34.

Harris P (2003) 'Am I alone in this grief?' User support for transracially adopted and fostered young people. In Argent H (ed.) *Models of Adoption Support.* BAAF, London.

Harris P (2005) 'Family is family . . . it does affect everybody in the family': Black relatives and adoption support. *Adoption and Fostering* **29(2)**: 66–75.

Hart A and Thomas H (2000) Controversial attachments: The indirect treatment of fostered and adopted children via Parent Co-Therapy. *Attachment and Human Development* **2(3)**: 306–27.

Hendry A and Vincent J (2002) Supporting adoptive families: An interagency response. *Representing Children* **8(2)**.

Hill C and Thompson M (2003) Mental and physical health co-morbidity. *Clinical Child Psychology and Psychiatry* **8(3)**: 315–21.

Hodges J, Steele M, Hillman S, Henderson K and Kaniuk J (2003) Changes in attachment representations over the first year of adoptive placement: Narratives of maltreated children. *Clinical Child Psychology and Psychiatry* **8(3)**: 351–67.

Howe D (1994) *On Being a Client.* Sage, London.

Howe D (1996a) *Adopters on Adoption.* BAAF, London.

Howe D (1996b) Adopters' relationships with their adopted children from adolescence to early adulthood. *Adoption and Fostering* **20(3)**: 35–43.

Howe D (1998) *Patterns of Adoption.* Blackwell, Oxford.

Howe D (2000) Attachment. In Horwath J (ed.) The *Child's World: Assessing children in need. The reader.* NSPCC, London.

Howe D (2003) Attachment disorders: Disinhibited attachment disorders and secure base distortions with special reference to adopted children. *Attachment and Human Development* **5(3)**: 265–70.

Howe D and Fearnley S (1999) Disorders of attachment and attachment therapy. *Adoption and Fostering* **23(2)**: 19–30.

Howe D and Fearnley S (2003) Disorders of attachment in adopted and fostered children: Recognition and treatment. *Clinical Child Psychology and Psychiatry* **8(3)**: 389–400.

Howe D and Steele M (2004) The implications of contact for maltreated children: Children traumatised by their contact experiences, and their adoptive parents' states of mind. In Neil, E and Howe D (eds) *Contact in Permanent Placements: Research, theory and practice.* BAAF, London.

Howe D, Brandon M, Hinings D and Schofield G (1999) *Attachment Theory, Child Maltreatment and Family Support.* Macmillan, London.

Hughes D (2003) Psychological interventions for the spectrum of attachment disorders and intrafamilial disorder. *Attachment and Human Development* **5(3)**: 271–7.

Hundleby M (1997) Open adoption. In Triseliotis J, Shireman J and Hundleby M, *Adoption: Theory, policy and practice.* Cassell, London.

Ivaldi G (2000) *Surveying Adoption: A comprehensive analysis of local authority adoptions 1998–1999 (England).* BAAF, London.

Jaffee B and Fanshel D (1970) *How They Fared in Adoption.* Child Welfare League of America, New York.

Jewett C (1995) *Helping Children Cope with Separation and Loss*, 2nd edn. BAAF/Batsford, London.

Jones D (2003) *Communicating with Vulnerable Children.* Department of Health, Royal College of Psychiatrists, London.

Joyce B (2003) Tools that dig deeper. *Community Care* 4 September.

Juffer F, Hoksbergen RAC, Riksen-Walraven JM and Kohnstamm GA (1997) Early intervention in adoptive families: Supporting maternal sensitive responsiveness, infant–mother attachment and infant competence. *Journal of Child Psychology and Psychiatry* **38**: 1039–50.

Kaniuk J (1992) The use of relationship in the preparation and support of adopters. *Adoption and Fostering* **16(2)**: 47–52.

Kelly C, Allan S, Roscoe P and Herrick E (2003) The Mental Health Needs of Looked After Children: An integrated multi-agency model of care. *Clinical Child Psychology and Psychiatry* **8(3)**: 323–35.

Kirton D and Wooger D (1999) *Experiences of Transracial Adoption.* BAAF, London.

Lanyando M (2003) The emotional tasks of moving from fostering to adoption: Transitions, attachment, separation and loss. *Clinical Child Psychology and Psychiatry* **8(3)**: 337–49.

Lowe N (1997) The changing face of adoption: The gist/donation model versus the contract services model. *Child and Family Law Quarterly* **9(4)**: 371–86.

Lowe N (2000) English adoption law: Past, present and future. In Katz S, Eekelaar J and Maclean M (eds) *Cross-currents: Family law and policy in the US and England.* Oxford University Press, Oxford.

Lowe N and Murch M (2002) *The Plan for the Child: Adoption or long-term fostering.* BAAF, London.

Lowe N, Murch M, Borkowski M, Weaver A and Beckford V with Thomas C (1999) *Supporting Adoption: Reframing the approach.* BAAF, London.

Lyons-Ruth K (1996) Attachment relationships among children with aggressive behaviour problems: The role of disorganised early attachment patterns. *Journal of Consulting and Clinical Psychology* **64**: 64–73.

Macaskill C (1991) The abused child in the substitute family: The family's perspective. In Batty D (ed.) *Sexually Abused Children.* BAAF, London.

Macaskill C (2002) *Safe Contact: Children in permanent placement and contact with their birth relatives.* Russell House, Lyme Regis, UK.

McCarthy G, Janeway J and Geddes A (2003) The impact of emotional and behavioural problems on the lives of children growing up in the care system. *Adoption and Fostering* **23(3)**: 14–19.

McNamara J (ed.) (1995) *Bruised before Birth.* BAAF, London.

McWhinnie AM (1967) *Adopted Children: How they grow up.* Routledge and Kegan Paul, London.

Magagna J (2003) Clinical concepts and caregiving contexts. In Archer C and Burnell A (eds) *Trauma, Attachment and Family Permanence.* Jessica Kingsley, London.

Mason K, Selman P and Hughes M (1999) Permanency planning for children with Down's Syndrome: The adolescent years. *Adoption and Fostering* **23(1)**: 31–9.

Masson J, Harrison C and Pavlovic A (1997) *Working with Children and 'Lost' Parents: Putting partnership into practice.* York Publishing Services, York, UK.

Mather M (2003) Health and adoption support. In Argent H (ed.) *Models of Adoption Support.* BAAF, London.

Meltzer H, Gatward R, Goodman R and Ford T (2000) *The Mental Health of Children and Adolescents in Great Britain.* Office for National Statistics, London.

Milham S, Bullock R, Hosie K and Haak M (1986) *Lost in Care: The problems of maintaining links between children in care and their families.* Gower, Aldershot, UK.

Monck E, Reynolds J and Wigfall V (2003) The Role of Concurrent Planning: making permanent placements of young children. BAAF, London.

Morris A (1999) *The Adoption Experience.* BAAF, London.

Myeroff R, Mertlich G and Gross J (1999) Comparative effectiveness of holding therapy with aggressive children. *Child Psychiatry and Human Development* **29**: 303–13.

Neil E (2002) Contact after adoption: The role of the agencies in making and supporting plans. *Adoption and Fostering* **26(1)**: 25–38.

Neil E (2003) Accepting the reality of adoption: Birth relatives' experiences of face-to-face contact. *Adoption and Fostering* **27(2)**: 32–43.

O'Connor T and Zeanah C (2003) Attachment disorders: Assessment strategies and treatment approaches. *Attachment and Human Development* **5(3)**: 321–6.

O'Neil C (2003) The simplicity and complexity of support. In Argent H (ed.) *Models of Adoption Support*. BAAF, London.

Owusu-Bempah J and Howitt D (1997) Socio-genealogical connectedness, attachment theory and child care practice. *Child and Family Social Work* **2**: 199–207.

Pallett C, Scott C, Blackeby K, Yule W and Weissman R (2002) Fostering changes: A cognitive-behavioural approach to helping foster parents manage children. *Adoption and Fostering* **26(1)**: 39–48.

Performance and Innovation Unit (2000) *The Prime Minister's Review of Adoption*. The Cabinet Office, London.

Piccinelli M, Tessari E, Bortolomasi M, Piasere O, Semenzin M, Garzotto N and Tansella M (1997) Efficacy of the alcohol use disorders identification test as a screening tool for hazardous alcohol intake and related disorders in primary care: A validity study. *British Medical Journal* **514**: 420–4.

Pinderhughes EE and Rosenberg KF (1990) Family-bonding with high risk placements: A therapy model that promotes the process of becoming a family. In Glidden LM (ed.) *Formed Families: Adoption of children with handicaps*. Haworth Press, New York.

Pitcher D (2002) Placement with grandparents: The issues for grandparents who care for their grandchildren. *Adoption and Fostering* **26(1)**: 6–14.

Prevatt Goldstein B and Spencer M (2000) *Race and Ethnicity*. BAAF, London.

Prior M (2003) Adoption support from an education adviser. In Argent H (ed.) *Models of Adoption Support*. BAAF, London.

Prior V and Glaser D (2006) Understanding attachment and attachment disorders – theory, evidence and practice. Jessica Kingsley, London.

Quinton D and Rutter M (1988) *Parenting Breakdown: The making and breaking of inter-generational links*. Avebury, Aldershot, UK.

Quinton D and Selwyn J (2006) Adoption in the UK. In McCauley C, Pecora P and Rose W (eds) *Enhancing the Wellbeing of Children and Families through Effective Interventions* Jessica Kingsley, London.

Quinton D, Rushton A, Dance C and Mayes D (1998) *Joining New Families: A study of adoption and fostering in middle childhood*. Wiley and Sons, Chichester.

Rashid SP (2000) The strengths of black families. *Adoption and Fostering* **24(1)**: 15–22.

Raynor L (1980) *The Adopted Child Comes of Age*. George Allen and Unwin, London.

Richards A and Ince L (2000) *Overcoming Obstacles: Looked After Children – Quality services for black and ethnic minority children and their families*. Family Rights Group, London.

Robson K and Savage A (2001) Assessing adult attachment: An interview course with Patricia Crittenden. *Child Abuse Review* **10(6)**: 440–8.

Rushton A (2003a) *Support for adoptive families: A review of current evidence on problems, needs and effectiveness. Adoption and Fostering* **27(3)**: 41–50.

Rushton A (2003b) Local authority and voluntary adoption agencies' arrangements for supporting adoptive families: A survey of UK practice. *Adoption and Fostering* **27(3)**: 51–60.

Rushton A (2004) A scoping and scanning review of research on the adoption of children placed from public care. *Clinical Child Psychology and Psychiatry* **9(1)**: 89–106.

Rushton A and Dance C (2003) *Adoption Support Services for Families in Difficulty*. BAAF, London.

Rushton A and Dance C (2004) Outcomes of late-placed adoptions: The adolescent years. *Adoption and Fostering* **28(1)**: 49–58.

Rushton A, Dance C, Quinton D and Mayes D (2001) *Siblings in Late Permanent Placements*. BAAF, London.

Rushton A, Mayes D, Dance C and Quinton D (2003) Parenting Late-Placed Children: The development of new relationships and the challenge of behavioural problems. *Clinical Child Psychology and Psychiatry* **8(3)**: 389–400.

Rustin M (2005) Conceptual analysis of critical moments in Victoria Climbie's life. *Child and Family Social Work* **10(1)**: 11–19.

Rutter M and the ERA Study Team (1998a) Developmental catch-up and deficit following adoption after marked early privation. *Journal of Child Psychology and Psychiatry* **39(4)**: 465–76.

Rutter M, Giller H and Hagell A (1998b) *Antisocial Behaviour by Young People*. Cambridge University Press, New York.

Rutter M, Kreppner J, O'Connor TG and the ERA Study Team (2001) Specificity and heterogeneity in children's responses to profound privation. *British Journal of Psychiatry* **179**: 97–103.

Ryan T and Walker R (1999) *Life Story Work*, 2nd edn. BAAF, London.

Salter AN (2002) *The Adopter's Handbook*. BAAF, London.

Schofield G (1998) Making sense of the ascertainable wishes and feelings of insecurely attached children. *Child and Family Law Quarterly* **10(4)**: 363–75.

Schofield G (2005) The voice of children in family placement decision-making: A developmental model. *Adoption and Fostering* **29(1)**: 29–44.

Schofield G, Beek M, Sargent K with Thoburn J (2000) *Growing Up in Foster Care*. BAAF, London.

Scott S and Lindsey C (2003) Therapeutic approaches in adoption. In Argent H (ed.) *Models of Adoption Support*. BAAF, London.

Scott S, Spender Q, Doolan M, Jacobs B and Aspland H (2001) Multicentre controlled trial of parenting groups for child antisocial behaviour in clinical practice. *British Medical Journal* **323**: 194–7.

Sellick C and Howell D (2003) *Innovative, Tried and Tested: A review of good practice in fostering*. Social Care Institute for Excellence, London.

Sellick C, Thoburn J and Philpot T (2004) *What Works in Adoption and Foster Care?* Barnados, Barkingside, UK.

Selwyn J and Quinton D (2004) Stability, permanence, outcomes and support: Foster care and adoption compared. *Adoption and Fostering* **28(4)**: 6–15.

Sinclair I (2002) *Causes of Foster Care Breakdown: Report on project commissioned for the parenting initiative*. Department of Health, London.

Sinclair I, Gibbs I and Wilson K (2004a) *Foster Carers: Why they stay and why they leave*. Jessica Kingsley, London.

Sinclair I, Wilson K and Gibbs I (2004b) *Foster Placements: Why they succeed and why they fail*. Jessica Kingsley, London.

Skuse D, Bentovim A, Hodges J, Stevenson J, Adreou C, Layando M, New M, Williams B and McMillan D (1998) Risk factors for development of sexually abusive behaviour in sexually victimised adolescent boys: Cross-sectional study. *British Medical Journal* **317(7152)**: 175–9.

Snaith R, Constantopoulos A, Jardine M and McGuffin P (1978) A clinical scale for the self-assessment of irritability. *British Journal of Psychiatry* **132**: 163–71.

Spangler G and Grossmann C (1993) Biobehavioural organisation in securely and insecurely attached infants. *Child Development* **64**: 1429–50.

Stalker K and Connors C (2003) Communicating with disabled children. *Adoption and Fostering* **27(1)**: 26–35.

Stams G-JJ, Juffer F, Rispens J and Hokbergen RAC (2001) The development and adjustment of 7-year-old children adopted in infancy. *Journal of Child Psychology and Psychiatry* **41(8)**: 1025–37.

Steele M, Hodges J, Kaniuk J, Hillman S and Henderson K (2003) Attachment representations and adoption: Associations between maternal states of mind and emotion narratives in previously maltreated children. *Journal of Child Psychotherapy* **29(2)**: 187–205.

Stovall KC and Dozier M (1998) Infants in foster care: An attachment perspective. *Adoption Quarterly* **2(1)**: 55–87.

Sykes M (2000) Adoption with contact: A study of adoptive parents and the impact of continuing contact with families of origin. *Adoption and Fostering* **24(2)**: 20–32.

Thoburn J (1990) *Success and Failure in Permanent Family Placement*. Avebury, Aldershot, UK.

Thoburn J, Norford L and Rashid S (2000) *Permanent Family Placement for Children of Minority Ethnic Origin*. Jessica Kingsley, London.

Thomas C, Beckford V, Lowe N and Murch M (1999) *Adopted Children Speaking*. BAAF, London.

Tingle N (1994) Grandparents speak. In Argent H (ed.) *See You Soon: Contact with children looked after by local authorities*. BAAF, London.

Triseliotis J (1973) *In Search of Origins*. Routledge and Kegan Paul, London.

Triseliotis J, Shireman J and Hundleby M (1997) *Adoption: Theory, policy and practice*. Cassell, London.

Turnpenny P (1995) *Secrets in the Genes: Adoption, inheritance and genetic disease*. BAAF, London.

Van Gulden H and Bartels-Rabb L (1995) *Real Parents, Real Children*. BAAF, London.

Ward P (2004) Achieving permanence for Looked After Children through special guardianship: A study of the experience of New Zealand guardians with implications for special guardianship in England. *Adoption and Fostering* **28(4)**: 16–27.

Williams L (2003) Online adoptions support and advice. In Argent H (cd.) *Models of Adoption Support*. BAAF, London.

Index